Looking Forward . . .

The Speech and Swallowing Guidebook for People with Cancer of the Larynx or Tongue

Fourth Edition

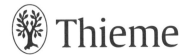

Looking Forward . . .

The Speech and Swallowing Guidebook for People with Cancer of the Larynx or Tongue

Fourth Edition

Jack E. Thomas, M.S., C.C.C.-S.L.P.
Supervisor
Division of Speech Pathology
Department of Neurology
Mayo Clinic
Rochester, Minnesota

Robert L. Keith, M.S., C.C.C.-S.L.P.
Associate (Emeritus)
Division of Speech Pathology
Mayo Clinic
Associate Professor (Emeritus)
Mayo Medical School
Rochester, Minnesota

Thieme Medical Publishers
New York • Stuttgart

Thieme New York
333 Seventh Avenue
New York, NY 10001
Consulting Medical Editor: Esther Gumpert
Associate Editor: J. Owen Zurhellen
Vice President, Production and Electronic Publishing: Anne T. Vinnicombe
Production Editor: Erik I. Wenskus
Marketing Director: Phyllis Gold
Director of Sales: Ross Lumpkin
Chief Financial Officer: Peter van Woerden
President: Brian D. Scanlan
Compositor: Thomson Press (India) Limited
Printer: The Maple-Vail Book Manufacturing Group

Library of Congress Cataloging in Publication Data is available from the publisher
Thomas, Jack E.
    Looking forward-- : the speech and swallowing guidebook for people
with cancer of the larynx or tongue / Jack E. Thomas, Robert L. Keith.— 4th ed.
      p. ; cm.
    Rev. ed. of: Looking forward-- / Robert L. Keith. 3rd ed. 1995.
    Includes index.
    ISBN 1-58890-294-3 (alk. paper) -- ISBN 3-13-666204-0 (alk. paper)
   1. Neck—Cancer—Popular works. 2. Mouth—Cancer—Popular works. 3. Laryngectomy—
Popular works. 4. Tongue—Surgery—Popular works. 5. Esophageal speech—Popular works.
6. Speech therapy—Popular works.
    [DNLM: 1. Laryngectomy—rehabilitation—Popular Works. 2. Adaptation, Psychological—
Popular Works. 3. Laryngeal Neoplasms—surgery—Popular Works. WV 540 T458L 2005]
I. Keith, Robert L. II. Title.
   RC280.N35T467 2005
   616.99'42206—dc22

Important note: Medical knowledge is ever-changing. As new research and clinical experience
broaden our knowledge, changes in treatment and drug therapy may be required. The authors
and editors of the material herein have consulted sources believed to be reliable in their efforts
to provide information that is complete and in accord with the standards accepted at the time
of publication. However, in view of the possibility of human error by the authors, editors, or
publisher of the work herein or changes in medical knowledge, neither the authors, editors, or
publisher, nor any other party who has been involved in the preparation of this work, warrants
that the information contained herein is in every respect accurate or complete, and they are not
responsible for any errors or omissions or for the results obtained from use of such information.
Readers are encouraged to confirm the information contained herein with other sources. For
example, readers are advised to check the product information sheet included in the package
of each drug they plan to administer to be certain that the information contained in this
publication is accurate and that changes have not been made in the recommended dose or in
the contraindications for administration. This recommendation is of particular importance in
connection with new or infrequently used drugs.

Some of the product names, patents, and registered designs referred to in this book are in fact
registered trademarks or proprietary names even though specific reference to this fact is not
always made in the text. Therefore, the appearance of a name without designation as
proprietary is not to be construed as a representation by the publisher that it is in the public
domain.

Printed in the United States of America

5 4 3 2 1

TNY ISBN 1-58890-294-3

GTV ISBN 3-13-666204-0

This book is dedicated to the many patients who have had head and neck cancer and members of their families whose invaluable insights, questions, and suggestions helped us write the first edition and subsequent revisions of *Looking Forward...* and to J.E.T.'s wife, Linda, and son, Loren, for their love and patience, and to R.L.K.'s wife, Lorraine, for her art and editing.

Contents

Preface

This guidebook is for people who have cancer of the mouth, tongue, larynx, or throat—the main structures responsible for speech and swallowing. Ideally, before you receive medical treatment or speech and swallowing therapy, you and your family will have an opportunity to read sections of *Looking Forward…: The Guidebook to Speech and Swallowing for People with Cancer of the Larynx or Tongue.* However, you may find much of the information helpful any time during your treatment and even after completion of treatment.

Over the years we, as speech pathologists, have provided speech and swallowing therapy to hundreds of people with cancer of the larynx, tongue, and related areas. Many have told us how much they have appreciated our help. At the same time, they have taught us a great deal as we helped them navigate through their course of cancer treatments. We've learned some important lessons: *no two persons with head and neck cancer are exactly alike.* What is true or best for one person may not be for another. The location and extent of disease in each person is different, and each person responds differently to cancer treatments and rehabilitation. And, when people hear and read new information about emotional and frightening topics, they often must hear and read it several times before they fully understand it. We hope *Looking Forward…* helps fill in the gaps when it is impossible to take in all the information provided by medical personnel and when it's difficult to think of the questions to ask when meeting with the professionals who can answer them.

Because of such individual and varied outcomes, in *Looking Forward…* we will not tell you exactly what you need to do, exactly what you will experience, or what you will feel during and after treatments or therapy for laryngeal, tongue, and related cancers. We have made an effort to avoid the use of words such as "always," "must," "should," and "never." Instead, we have tried to use words such as "may," "generally," "sometimes," "usually," and "often." Our aim is to provide you with accurate, basic information about treatments for cancer of the mouth and throat—radiation therapy, chemotherapy, and surgery—and therapy for the speech and swallowing impairments caused by cancer and cancer-fighting treatments. At the same time we realize that rehabilitation after head and neck cancer goes beyond therapy for speech and swallowing. Rather, rehabilitation is about communicating while working, playing, relating with friends and loved ones, coping with dramatic changes in one's life, and being hopeful about the future. We hope we have captured some of this, as well.

For specific information about your disease, treatment options, course of recovery, and speech and swallowing rehabilitation, you will need to ask questions. Ask your physicians. Ask your speech pathologist. Ask your other caregivers. No question is unimportant. We suggest that you use the designated space in each section of this book to write your questions and concerns, and then discuss them with your health care team. Use the same space to take notes. When you read an unfamiliar word printed in *italics,* look it up in the glossary at the end of the book. Also, to help you better understand your medical condition, ask your physician to sketch in the area of your cancer involvement using the illustrations at the end of Chapter 3.

One final note: every medical institution has its own policies and protocols. The approaches, procedures, equipment, and other aspects of care practiced at the institution where you receive your care may vary from those described in this book.

Acknowledgments

Robert L. Keith, M.S, C.C.C., a speech pathologist at the Mayo Clinic, Rochester, Minnesota, for over four decades, developed the original concept of this book. Mr. Keith treated many laryngectomized people, before and after their surgeries. He kept a log of their questions, and it became clear that the same questions came up again and again. These questions and their answers were compiled and sent to former patients and their spouses for their review. The results of that project developed into the first edition of *Looking Forward... A Guidebook for the Laryngectomee.* Mr. Keith was assisted by Candice May, a medical communications specialist and developer of patient education materials at Mayo Clinic-Rochester. Other experts were consulted: Harvey L.C. Coates, M.B., F.R.C.S.; Kenneth D. Devine, M.D.; Howard Shane, Ph.D.; Ruby C. Flaaten, R.N.; Nancy Roberts, R.N.; Ann Schutt, M.D.; Bruce W. Pearson, M.D.; David Hartman, Ph.D.; and John W. Desley, Medical Illustrator.

The second and third editions of *Looking Forward...* were written by Robert L. Keith and included updates and additional information. Those editions have been translated into Spanish, French, German, Dutch, and Turkish.

This fourth edition of the book is a collaboration between Jack E. Thomas, M.S., C.C.C.-S.P., and Mr. Keith, colleagues in Speech Pathology at the Mayo Clinic for over 20 years. The title of this book, *Looking Forward... The Speech and Swallowing Guidebook for People with Cancer of the Larynx or Tongue,* and the content have changed to better reflect our clinical practice and that of speech pathologists nationwide, as well as the experiences of our patients.

Many esteemed colleagues at the Mayo Clinic-Rochester have made important contributions to this fourth edition. Our sincere thanks to Robert E. Foote, M.D., Department of Radiation Oncology, for information on the role of radiation therapy in the treatment of head and neck cancer; Jean Girardi, P.T., Department of Physical Medicine and Rehabilitation, for information on physical therapy and home exercises after head and neck cancer treatments; Scott Okuno, M.D., Department of Medical Oncology, for information on the use of chemotherapy for head and neck cancer; and Adele Pattinson, R.D, L.D., CNSD, Department of Clinical Dietetics, for information on enteral feeding.

1

The Diagnosis of Cancer of the Larynx or Tongue

- ◆ **Signs and Symptoms**
- ◆ **Head and Neck Examination**
  - Oral Cavity
  - Indirect Laryngoscopy
  - Fiberoptic Laryngoscopy
  - Lymph Gland Inspection of the Neck
- ◆ **Radiological Imaging Tests**
- ◆ **Physical Examination before Biopsy**
- ◆ **Direct Laryngoscopy and Biopsy**

◆ Signs and Symptoms

As you may know, there are several signs and symptoms of cancer of the *larynx*, also known as *laryngeal* cancer. You have undoubtedly experienced some of them. Perhaps your voice has sounded hoarse for quite some time. It may be difficult for you to swallow—occasionally even painful. Some people notice a burning sensation when they swallow hot foods or acidic liquids such as orange juice. Others have an aching in one ear, which is caused by "*referred pain*" from the *tumor*. This happens because nerves in the larynx connect with nerves in the ear region and "refer" or send pain from the larynx to the ear. Sometimes, the first symptom of laryngeal cancer is the coughing up of blood, the appearance of a lump in the neck, difficulty with breathing, or frequent throat clearing or a persistent cough.

These signs and symptoms, whether they appear together or separately, suggest to the *otolaryngologist* the possibility of a tumor in the area or around the larynx. The exact nature of these symptoms, however, can be determined only after a thorough head and neck examination. This may include examining the oral cavity (all aspects of the mouth), *indirect laryngoscopy*, *fiberoptic laryngoscopy*, lymph gland inspection (inspecting and feeling the neck), radiological imaging (to be described later), and a *biopsy* during *direct laryngoscopy*. These procedures are described in the following text.

◆ Head and Neck Examination

Oral Cavity

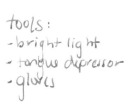

The head and neck examination starts with examination of the lips and the oral cavity (mouth). It requires a bright light and a tongue depressor. The physician looks at all aspects of the mouth including the lips, teeth, gums, the space between the teeth and gums, the roof of the mouth, the floor of the mouth, the cheeks, the salivary glands, the tongue, and the back of the throat. The physician wears gloves and uses a finger to look for sores and to feel the tongue and other parts of the mouth to help detect lumps, swelling, color changes, or anything unusual.

Oral cancer is commonly found on the front and side of the tongue and the floor of the mouth. It occurs about half as often as laryngeal cancer. People who are more likely to get oral cancer are those who smoke, those who use chewing tobacco, and those who drink alcohol. Cancer of the lip is most common in people who are exposed to large amounts of sunlight. Cancer of the oropharynx, the tongue base, and the tonsil is one of the areas of cancer that seems to be increasing in occurrence.

Indirect Laryngoscopy

By now, your physician has probably already examined your larynx using a method called indirect laryngoscopy (Fig. **1–1**). In this procedure, a small hand-held mirror is inserted into the back of the mouth. The physician then reflects a light onto the mirror by way of a second mirror located at his or her forehead. This is a quick and easy technique, although the mirror in the mouth can cause some people to gag. Sometimes the physician will use an anesthetic spray to reduce gagging.

With this method, the physician can determine the movement of the *vocal folds*, identify growths on the vocal folds and the upper part of the throat, and view the back part of the tongue.

Fiberoptic Laryngoscopy

Another technique for viewing the vocal folds and surrounding structures is *fiberoptic endoscopy* or fiberoptic laryngoscopy. After spraying the inside of the nose with an anesthetic, the physician inserts a thin, flexible, tubelike scope through the nasal passage down to the level of the larynx. With this method, the physician can view the entire nasal area, throat, and larynx. Sometimes a camera is connected to the scope to take photographs or record the movement of structures, including the larynx. The physician is primarily looking for signs of disease all along this route. If areas of concern are noted, such as a tumor growing into the vocal folds, additional tests are required because it is important to identify and treat disease sooner rather than later.

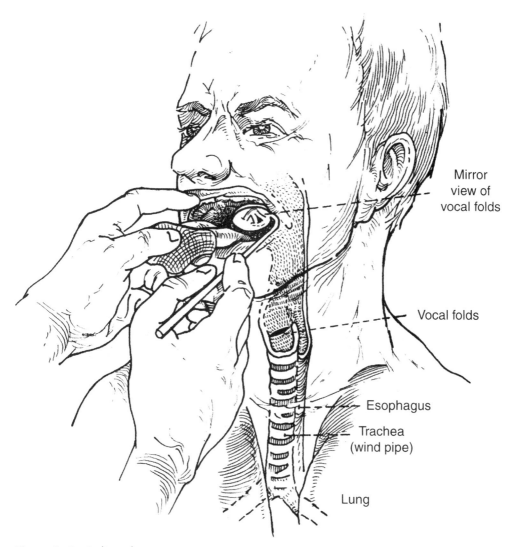

Figure 1–1 Indirect laryngoscopy.

Lymph Gland Inspection of the Neck

Thorough inspection of the lymph glands in the neck is an important part of ~~spreads to the lymph nodes first.~~ the head and neck examination (Fig. **1–2**). Your physician does this because when a tumor in the larynx or tongue spreads, it usually first travels to the *lymph nodes* in the neck. After inspecting your neck from the front, the physician may stand behind you and use his or her fingers to feel the sides and front of the neck and under the chin to detect any enlarged neck nodes. The physician may ask you about any lumps you are aware of in your neck. If there is concern that a lump may be *malignant,* a special syringe and needle may be used to remove some cells from the lump for examination. This test is called *fine-needle biopsy* or *fine-needle aspiration.*

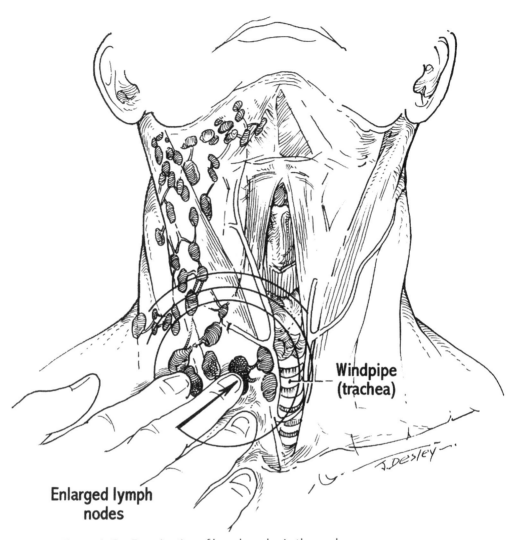

Windpipe (trachea)

Enlarged lymph nodes

Figure 1–2   Examination of lymph nodes in the neck.

◆ Radiological Imaging Tests

In a complete head and neck examination, your physician will order radiological imaging tests. X-rays of the neck can give some information about the airway and changes in soft tissue. X-rays may be taken of the lungs to ensure they are clear of disease. Computed tomography *(CT scan or CT scanning)* is a primary way of imaging the larynx (Fig. **1–3**). CT is particularly good at showing the size of a malignant tumor and the extent of its growth. *Magnetic resonance imaging* (MRI) may be used to help determine the spread of a tumor. For CT scanning and MRI, the patient passes through a doughnut-shaped machine. There is no pain associated with these tests, but some people say they feel

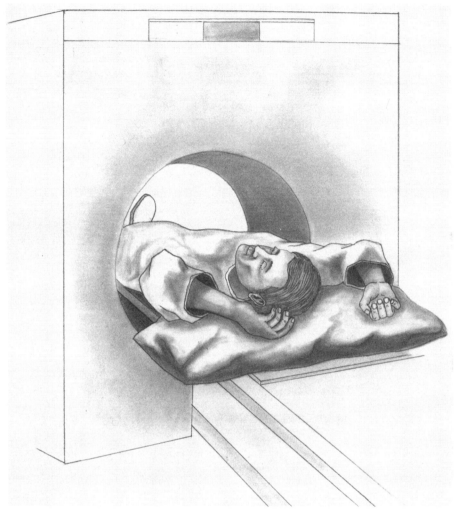

Figure 1–3 Computed tomography (CT) or magnetic resonance imaging (MRI) machine.

closed-in during the procedure. The physician or technician performing the tests will be sensitive to this and make suggestions on how to be most comfortable during these tests. In addition, your physician may decide other radiological tests are necessary to evaluate the tumor's extent.

◆ Physical Examination before Biopsy

If the oral examination, indirect laryngoscopy, fiberoptic laryngoscopy, and radiological studies indicate that a tumor is present, your physician will need to perform another test before deciding how to proceed. The final diagnosis *need anesthesia?*

physical exam

then

a biopsy!

can be made only after a biopsy has been done. Often a biopsy can be performed in the doctor's office. If general anesthesia is necessary for the biopsy, your physician will schedule you for a physical examination. This includes reviewing your medical history and asking about the medical history of your family members, checking your vital signs (temperature, blood pressure, pulse), taking blood and urine samples, testing your heart and lungs, asking about the medications you are taking, and more. The physician who performs this examination will inform your other physicians whether you appear to be well enough to undergo anesthesia.

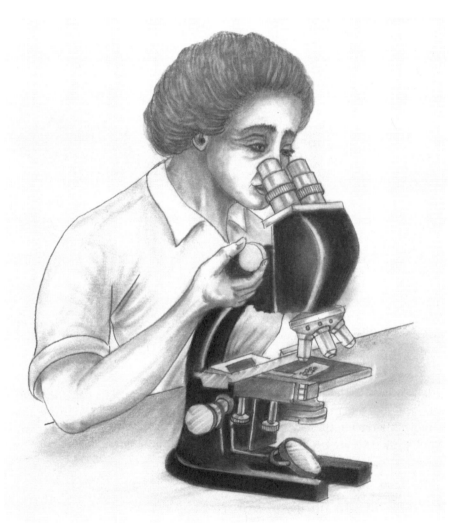

Figure 1–4   A pathologist examines a thin slice of tissue for cancer cells.

◆ Direct Laryngoscopy and Biopsy

When the biopsy of the larynx and surrounding areas is performed during direct laryngoscopy while you are anesthetized, you will not feel any discomfort. To perform this biopsy, the physician uses a tubelike instrument with a light and a magnifying lens on one end. This instrument is called a *laryngoscope*. It is placed inside the mouth and down into the throat. By looking through one end of the laryngoscope, the physician can see directly into the larynx. A piece of tissue is removed from the area where the other tests have indicated a tumor is growing. Then this tissue is sliced into very thin sections and examined under a microscope by a *pathologist*—a physician who specializes in diagnosing disease by microscopic examination of the cells (Fig. **1–4**). If there is only a small spot of concern on the vocal folds or other parts of the larynx, it may be possible for the physician to completely remove the diseased tissue during direct laryngoscopy. If disease has replaced most of the normal tissue of the vocal folds or surrounding area, however, you will need other lifesaving treatments.

2

Normal Anatomy of the Head and Neck for Breathing, Swallowing, and Speech

This chapter describes the normal anatomy and physiology (body parts and how they function) of the mouth and throat for breathing, swallowing, and speaking, and how they are affected by cancer and the medical treatments to cure it.

A simplified illustration of the anatomy of the mouth and throat for breathing, swallowing, and speech is shown in Fig. **2–1**. The air you breathe enters through the nose and mouth. It then passes through the *oropharynx,* which is just behind the tongue at the back of the throat. At this point the throat is still a common pathway for both food and air. After air passes the oropharynx it comes to the *epiglottis* and then moves through the *false vocal folds* and the true vocal folds. These are the main parts of the larynx. From there, air moves down through the trachea (windpipe) and into the lungs.

The larynx functions as a valve to prevent food from entering the trachea. It closes off the entryway to the trachea. This is very important. If food or liquids enter the airway (aspiration), *pulmonary* (lung) problems such as pneumonia may result.

When food is swallowed, it starts out on the same pathway as air for breathing. The lips keep food in the mouth and the tongue moves the food around while it is being chewed in preparation for swallowing. Saliva moistens the food and begins to break it down for digestion. The tongue moves the food to the back of the mouth (Fig. **2–2**) and, during the swallow, the food passes through the oropharynx and then downward (Fig. **2–3**). Then the path changes. The epiglottis tilts down. The false vocal folds and true vocal folds close tightly and rise up and under the back of the tongue. (In front of a mirror, watch your Adam's apple move upward when you swallow saliva.) This action channels the food away from the larynx and airway. The pharyngeal constrictor muscles move the food down through the *pharynx* with a squeezing, wavelike movement into the *esophagus* (Fig. **2–4**), and the esophagus takes the food to the stomach.

Another function of the larynx is the production of voice for speech. Air passing up from the lungs during exhalation (breathing out) and through the larynx causes the vocal folds to vibrate. This vibration creates a sound. Did you ever place a blade of grass between your thumbs and blow on it to make a sound? The reason you could make a noise with a blade of grass is essentially the same as the reason sound can be produced with the larynx. Air causes the

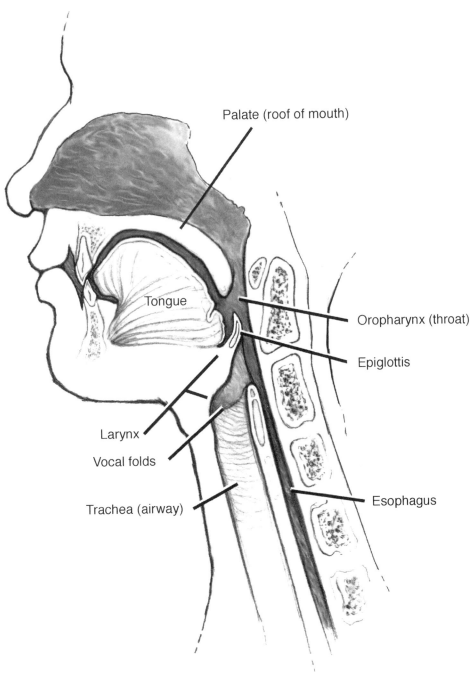

Palate (roof of mouth)

Tongue

Oropharynx (throat)

Epiglottis

Larynx

Vocal folds

Trachea (airway)

Esophagus

Figure 2–1   A simplified illustration of the mouth and throat for breathing, swallowing, and speech. (Used with permission of the Mayo Foundation for Medical Education and Research.)

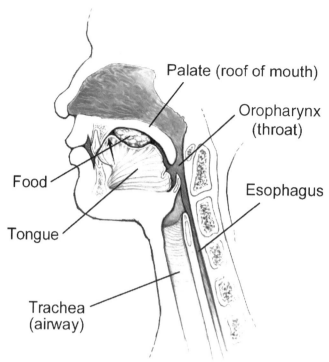

Figure 2–2 The tongue moves food to the back of the mouth in preparation for swallowing. (Used with permission of the Mayo Foundation for Medical Education and Research.)

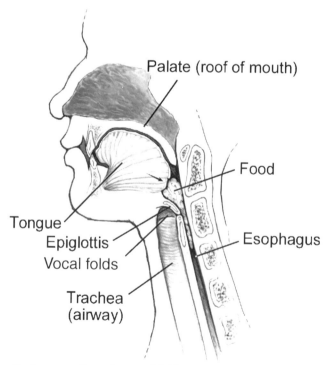

Figure 2–3 During a swallow, the vocal folds close and the larynx rises up to channel food away from the airway. (Used with permission of the Mayo Foundation for Medical Education and Research.)

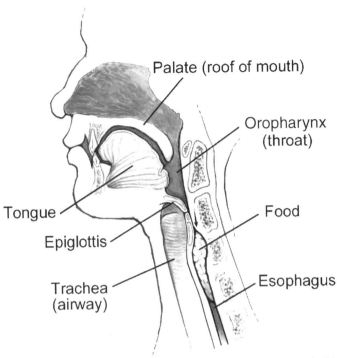

Figure 2–4　Food passes through the esophagus toward the stomach. (Used with permission of the Mayo Foundation for Medical Education and Research.)

blade of grass to vibrate. This, in turn, makes the air vibrate. The vibrating air produces the sound. When the vocal folds are set into vibration by air from the lungs, voice is produced. This voice is shaped into speech mainly by the tongue and lips. The actual process is quite complex, with many rapid, overlapping, and complicated movements, but this simplified explanation describes the basic processes of voice and speech production.

3

Treatments for Cancer of the Larynx or Tongue

◆ Members of Your Medical Team

◆ Important Questions to Ask

◆ Whatever Cancer Treatments You Decide Upon: Read This!

◆ Members of Your Medical Team

If your ear, nose, and throat (ENT) surgeon or otolaryngologist finds that you have cancer of the larynx or the tongue, or in the surrounding areas, other members of the medical team may be asked to also evaluate you and additional tests may be performed. A *radiation oncologist* can review the results of all your tests and determine if radiation therapy may be effective in treating your disease. A *medical oncologist* can decide if *chemotherapy* is appropriate for treating the disease. Your doctors will discuss the kinds of approaches that are available and what would be best for managing your disease. Sometimes a person with cancer of the larynx or tongue is advised to have only one form of treatment. Often, a combination of treatments is suggested, such as surgery first, followed by radiation therapy. Or radiation therapy may be recommended first, followed by surgery if the disease progresses. Sometimes chemotherapy may be recommended in combination with radiation therapy or surgery.

Other members of the medical team may meet with you, depending on your cancer and recommended treatment. A *speech pathologist* will evaluate your voice, speech, and swallowing ability and discuss with you and your family how surgery, radiation therapy, chemotherapy, or a combination of these treatments may affect them. A *dietitian* may meet with you if you have experienced weight loss or if the cancer treatments you receive require changing the consistency of your foods. A dentist or *maxillofacial prosthodontist* will examine your teeth and may start you on daily fluoride treatments to help preserve your teeth before, during, and after cancer treatments. A nurse who specializes in various cancer treatments may meet with you and instruct you in certain procedures. Other specialists and technicians may be involved.

◆ Important Questions to Ask

If you have cancer of the larynx, tongue, or other areas of the head and neck, the decisions you make about how to proceed will depend on your health, the extent of your cancer, an individualized discussion about the pros and cons of treatment, and what you decide is right for you. Depending on the extent and stage of the disease, this can be a very difficult decision, perhaps even a life-or-death decision. You and your family will need to ask some important questions:

- Where, exactly, is the cancer located?
- How fast is it growing? Is it spreading to other parts of my body?
- Is this life threatening?
- If I agree to a particular treatment, what are the prospects for cure?
- If I decide on surgery, how much of the affected area and the surrounding tissue will be removed, and how does the surgeon know how much is enough?
- Are there other kinds of treatment?
- How will each treatment affect the way I breathe? Swallow? Speak?
- Will the treatment be painful? How will pain be alleviated?
- How will my face and neck change in appearance?
- How long will it take before I have recovered to a level that is the maximum I can expect to achieve?
- How will it change my life?
- What are the potential short- and long-term complications of each treatment modality?
- What will happen if the proposed treatment does not work? What can be done then?
- What is my physician's personal experience with the recommended treatment?
- Is there someone I can talk with who has had similar disease and treatment?

To help you understand the location and extent of abnormal tissue in your larynx, tongue, or surrounding structures, ask your physician to draw in those areas using the illustrations in Fig. **3–1**.

◆ Whatever Cancer Treatments You Decide Upon: Read This!

Your physicians and other members of the health care team are the best sources for information about your disease. Every person is different, with a unique medical condition and life situation. Your physicians may refer you to

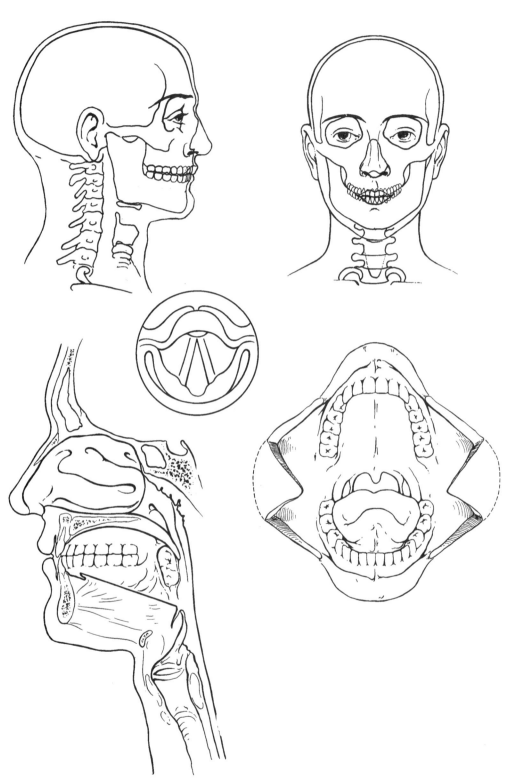

Figure 3–1 Ask your physician to draw in the areas of concern. (Used with permission of the Mayo Foundation for Medical Education and Research.)

Table 3–1 Records Checklist

Your name _____ Your birth date _____

Your cancer diagnosis_____ Date of your cancer diagnosis_____

Important laboratory and x-ray results _____

_____

_____

Information about your type(s) of cancer treatment

Radiation therapy

Part of body treated _____

Number of treatments _____

Dates of treatment _____

_____

Side effects _____

_____

_____

Chemotherapy

Drug names _____

_____

_____

_____

Number of treatments _____

Dates of treatment _____

_____

_____

Side effects _____

_____

_____

Surgery

Type of operation(s) _____

_____

Date(s) of operation(s) _____

Name of surgeon _____

Hospital _____

Other cancer treatment medications

Name of treatment(s) _____

_____

_____

_____

(Continued)

Table 3–1   (*Continued*)

Dates of treatment(s) _____

_____

_____

Location of treatment(s) _____

_____

_____

Complications _____

_____

Non – cancer treatment medications you've taken or you're taking

Names _____

_____

Doses _____

_____

Complications _____

_____

_____

Medical professionals who've participated in your care

Names and phone numbers _____

_____

_____

Used with permission of the Mayo Foundation for Medical Education and Research.

other sources of information on head and neck cancer and its treatment, such as publications from the American Cancer Society and the National Cancer Institute. You may decide to seek out a second medical opinion. Remember, there are many sources of medical information on the World Wide Web and other places. Be careful with "facts" you receive from sources other than from a physician who has examined you. Otherwise, you may be misled by information that does not pertain to your specific medical condition. If you find information that you do not understand or if it conflicts with information your medical team has given you, take that information to the physicians who know you. Ask questions and listen.

Additionally, whatever cancer treatment or treatments you choose, consider using the records checklist in Table **3–1**. It will help you keep track of important information about your diagnosis and conventional treatments (radiation therapy, chemotherapy, surgery) as well as complementary treatments such as nutrition and other approaches.

4

Radiation Therapy

◆ **Preparation for Radiation Therapy**

◆ **Possible Side Effects of Radiation Therapy**

◆ **Radiation Therapy Treatments**

Radiation therapy is used to destroy cancer cells. Radiation therapy is also known as "radiation," "radiotherapy," and "irradiation." Cells are most vulnerable to radiation therapy when they are dividing and growing. Because most cancer cells multiply at a faster rate than most normal cells, they are more susceptible to radiation therapy. This is why radiation therapy can usually destroy cancer cells. Healthy cells may become damaged by radiation therapy, but they can recover.

For early cancers confined to the vocal folds, the tongue, or related structures, your physician may recommend radiation therapy to treat the cancer. Surgery will be necessary if the cancer returns. For an explanation of what is considered an "early tumor," ask your physician.

Late or large tumors tend not to respond as well to radiation therapy. With these tumors, surgery is usually recommended first, followed by radiation therapy. Again, ask your physician for an explanation of "late tumors," what this means, and a description of any other treatment possibilities.

If radiation therapy is recommended to treat your cancer, the number of treatments, the total dose of radiation, and the schedule for receiving treatments will depend on the size and location of the cancer, your health, and any other treatments you are receiving or have received in the past. Sometimes radiation therapy is administered in conjunction with chemotherapy. Much depends on each person's individual situation.

As described in other sections of this book, before any treatment you may undergo an evaluation with a multispecialty team of physicians and other health care providers so that the treatment can be designed and planned for your individual situation.

◆ Preparation for Radiation Therapy

When you are treated with radiation therapy alone, or if it is combined with chemotherapy or surgery, the radiation therapy process begins with a planning session called a "simulation." Here are the typical steps in preparation for and undergoing radiation therapy for cancer of the larynx and surrounding areas.

During the radiation therapy simulation process, you will lie down on your back on a flat table. A plastic face mask is used to help you hold your head and neck still during the radiation treatment (Fig. **4–1**). The plastic face mask ensures that you are exactly in the same position each day for your treatment and that there is no movement during the treatment. This helps to make the radiation therapy more accurate and precise. To make the mask, a sheet of plastic is placed in a warm water bath until it becomes soft and flexible. Then it is draped over your face and a hair dryer is used to blow it dry. The mask hardens within just a few minutes. There are many holes in the plastic so that you can easily breathe and see through it.

Once the plastic mask has been made, the radiation oncologist takes some x-rays of the general area to be treated. Also, a computed tomography (CT) scan of the head and neck area is performed while you are lying on your back on a flat table with the face mask on. The radiation oncologist uses the x-rays and CT scan images to identify the cancer and the normal tissue. Individualized custom blocks are fabricated to aim and focus the radiation beams on the cancer while minimizing the dose of radiation therapy to the surrounding normal structures. After the radiation beams are determined, the blocks are fabricated, and the radiation dose calculations are performed, you are ready to begin your treatments. The simulation procedure takes an hour or two to complete.

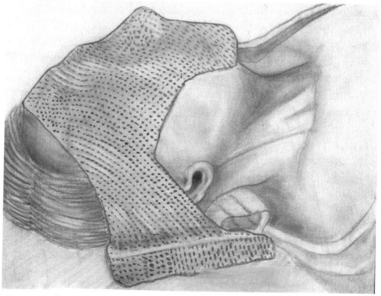

Figure 4–1   A plastic face mask helps to hold your head and neck still during radiation therapy treatments. The face mask has holes so you can see and breathe easily.

Tattoos the size of a small freckle or smaller may be placed on the skin of your neck to use as a treatment setup reference each day. These tattoos are permanent and prevent the inaccuracies of marking the treatment setup points with ink, which may smear or wash off. In most instances, these tattoos are tiny and not noticeable. Laser lights in the treatment room are used to line up the tattoos to ensure that you are on the table in the same position each day. Often these marks can be placed on the mask rather than tattooing the skin.

◆ Radiation Therapy Treatments

Typically, radiation treatments are administered on a daily basis, five days a week, Monday through Friday, with no treatments on weekends, for a six- to seven-week period. In some instances, two treatments are given each day during the entire course of treatment or during the last two or three weeks. Your radiation oncologist will determine what type of treatment will be most effective for you.

Radiation therapy treatments are administered through a *linear accelerator* (Fig. **4–2**). During each treatment, you lie on your back on a flat table with the face mask on. Highly skilled radiation therapists help the physician administer your treatment each day. Typically, it takes 15 or 20 minutes for

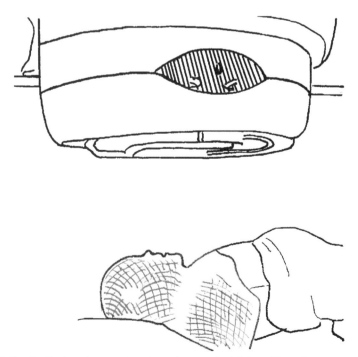

Figure 4–2   Radiation therapy treatments are administered by a linear accelerator.

each radiation treatment. You should plan on 30 to 45 minutes each day to take into account waiting for your turn, being set up for the treatment, receiving the treatment, and scheduling your next appointment.

Your radiation oncologist will meet with you on a regular basis to see how things are going with the treatment. These visits will include monitoring the response of the cancer to the radiation therapy and helping you manage any side effects related to it. You will also meet with nurses, dietitians, social workers, and other members of the health care team during the course of treatment to help with any concerns that might arise.

◆ Possible Side Effects of Radiation Therapy

The side effects of radiation therapy depend on the area treated with radiation therapy and the dose that is administered with each treatment. In general, during the first two or three weeks of radiation treatment, most people notice some minimal swelling of the face or neck, dry mouth, and altered taste. By the fifth or sixth week of treatment, these symptoms may develop into complete loss of taste, dry mouth with thick saliva, and painful mouth and throat sores. Your physician will recommend specific oral care and pain medicine to minimize discomfort, improve taste, and alleviate dryness. A salt and soda water mouth rinse and gargle may be soothing and promote healing. To make this mouth rinse, mix one-half teaspoon of baking soda and one-half teaspoon of salt with one cup of warm water. Swish this mixture inside your mouth and spit it out. Repeat swishing and spitting until you have used the entire amount. Do not swallow this solution. Over-the-counter products are available that coat and soothe your mouth and throat. Be certain to ask your radiation oncologist if these are right for you. It will be important that you avoid certain products, such as those with alcohol as an ingredient, which will cause further irritation.

Mouth sores may make chewing and swallowing some foods and liquids uncomfortable. Soft and moist foods may be more comfortable to eat. Spicy foods may be irritating, and hot or cold foods and liquids may become very uncomfortable. The mouth may become so sensitive that only a liquid diet can be tolerated. Typical medications for mouth and throat pain include Tylenol, Tylenol with codeine, morphine, and fentanyl. If the pain from mouth or throat sores limits your ability to eat and drink, a dietitian will help by suggesting liquid nutritional supplements. In some instances, it is necessary to place a feeding tube in the stomach to ensure that you receive enough fluid and nutrition during the course of radiation therapy (see Appendix C). This reduces the need for painful chewing or swallowing. Patients are able to maintain or gain weight and keep up their energy by using the feeding tube. They also heal more quickly once the radiation therapy has been completed.

Toward the end of the radiation therapy program, the skin in the neck area may turn red and may itch and burn. Special lotions, creams, and bandages will be given to you to help comfort and heal the skin. Once the course of radiation treatments has been completed, the skin usually heals quite rapidly. Within about two weeks it turns dark and dry like a suntan, and like a suntan it peels off and the skin lightens up again. By four or six weeks after completing the radiation therapy, the sores in the mouth and throat usually go away and you are able to eat more comfortably. Around three months after completing a course of radiation therapy, the sense of taste begins to return.

One of the potential permanent side effects of radiation therapy is a dry mouth. A dry mouth causes swallowing problems. You may find that it takes you longer to eat. You may need to take smaller bites and chew the food well before swallowing. A dry mouth may be prevented in some situations by limiting the dose of radiation therapy that the salivary glands receive, or alleviated by using medications such as Ethyol or Salagen. Acupuncture has been reported to help production of saliva for some people. If your mouth is permanently dry after radiation therapy, and if you do not have difficulty swallowing water, you may find the most simple and practical thing to do is to carry a plastic bottle of water with you at all times so that a sip of water is readily available. Some people find products such as artificial saliva helpful for adding moisture to the mouth; others find these products disappointing and the effects very temporary.

Radiation therapy can treat cancer. As with any treatment for eliminating life-threatening disease, however, it has some undesirable long-term consequences—it can affect speech, but it particularly affects swallowing. As cancers are destroyed by radiation therapy, particularly in people who have large and advanced cancers, scar tissue can form within the mouth or throat, including within the primary muscles that control swallowing—the pharyngeal constrictors. Because these muscles move food and liquids down the throat toward the stomach, when their movement becomes sluggish or diminished in any way, swallowing problems result. A person may develop permanent swallowing problems so severe a feeding tube may be required.

Swallowing problems are complex and may be due to many factors. The degree of swallowing difficulty each person experiences depends on the amount of radiation used, the locations where the radiation beams were directed, whether chemotherapy was part of the treatment, and the exact location where head and neck surgery was performed. Evaluation and treatment by a speech pathologist can be quite helpful to improve your swallowing ability. See Appendix D for information on swallowing after head and neck cancer treatments.

Saliva cleans and protects the teeth from decay. Because radiation therapy to the mouth and throat causes the salivary glands to stop working almost immediately, special fluoride dental treatments are necessary to preserve the teeth. You will see a dentist before starting the radiation therapy to check the condition of the teeth and to fabricate a "fluoride carrier." The fluoride carrier looks a lot like the mouth guard that athletes wear. The dentist will give you a gel containing fluoride and calcium to put in the fluoride carrier. You will place the carrier on your teeth for about five minutes or so every morning and every night. Brushing, flossing, using fluoride, and having your teeth cleaned will prevent the development of cavities in your teeth.

However, if the teeth are in poor condition prior to radiation therapy, the dentist will recommend removal of the teeth first. A most serious complication can occur when a tooth needs to be removed after radiation therapy. Because of the effects of radiation, sometimes the gums and/or bones do not heal. A person can develop an open socket that can become infected. Usually this infection can be treated with antibiotics and/or hyperbaric oxygen treatments, or it can be removed through minor surgery. Rarely, major surgery, including removal of a portion of the jawbone, is required to remove the infection. This serious complication can be prevented by removing any teeth in poor condition prior to beginning radiation therapy and by maintaining good dental health through brushing, flossing, dental cleanings, and fluoride treatments.

If the thyroid gland in the neck is within the radiation field, it may stop producing thyroid hormone. This condition, known as hypothyroidism, can cause symptoms such as lack of energy, a sensation of feeling cold all the time, constipation, dry skin, weight gain, and hair loss. You will be monitored closely for these symptoms and through blood tests. Hypothyroidism can be easily corrected by taking an inexpensive thyroid hormone pill every day.

If you are treated with radiation alone or with both surgery and radiation therapy, or radiation and chemotherapy, scar tissue may develop, particularly in the throat and neck. This can lead to stiffness and weakness of the neck, shoulder, and arm with pain and limited movement. These symptoms can be minimized by evaluation by a physical medicine and rehabilitation physician, who will give you some physical therapy exercises to perform.

If the ears are within the radiation field, dry wax may accumulate, but it can be removed by an ear, nose, and throat (*ENT*) physician. Because the eustachian tube that connects the middle ear to the back of the throat does not function as it did before radiation therapy, chronic serous otitis media (middle-ear infection) may develop. This condition may require placement of tubes through the eardrums to drain fluid. With high doses of radiation therapy, hearing loss due to nerve damage may result.

For men, if a portion of the face or chin is irradiated, you may find that you do not need to shave as often.

In summary, radiation therapy can cure some head and neck cancer, but side effects are common. Not all of the short- and long-term side effects of radiation therapy occur in each patient, and their severity, if they do occur, may vary from mild to severe. Side effects may be temporary or permanent. The incidence and severity of these side effects of radiation therapy depend on the area treated, the dose of radiation therapy you receive, and the addition of surgery or chemotherapy or both. Your radiation oncologist can answer your specific questions.

5

Chemotherapy

- ◆ **Preparation for Chemotherapy Treatments**
- ◆ **Chemotherapy Treatments**
- ◆ **Possible Side Effects of Chemotherapy**

Sometimes *chemotherapy* is used to treat the primary cancer or help keep cancer of the head and neck from spreading to other parts of the body. These powerful anticancer drugs may be combined with radiation and/or with surgery. Like radiation therapy, chemotherapy can affect healthy cells as well as kill cancer cells. Chemotherapy is generally used for advanced cancers.

Chemotherapy drugs for laryngeal and related cancers are usually delivered intravenously. The schedule for receiving chemotherapy and the amount received depends on the location and extent of the cancer and the type of chemotherapy drugs that are used. Some side effects of these drugs include nausea, loss of appetite, sores and sensitivity in the mouth, swelling and soreness in the throat, difficulty swallowing (all these can lead to loss of weight), fatigue, and hair loss. However, the type and severity of side effects vary from person to person. For example, some people experience few or mild unpleasant effects, whereas others may have a more severe response. Some people do not experience side effects of chemotherapy until they are near the conclusion of all their treatments, and most of the side effects go away soon after the treatments are finished.

If your physicians recommend chemotherapy, they may have already answered many of your questions. These are commonly asked questions about chemotherapy:

- What are the names of the chemotherapy drugs I will receive? (Ask the physician to write them down or spell them for you.)
- How do the drugs work?
- What kind of treatment is it? Intravenous? Pills?
- How many treatments will I receive and over what period of time?
- What are the prospects for a cure?
- What are the side effects of these drugs and can they be reduced?
- Do you have printed information I can read about the chemotherapy I need?
- Are there other sources of information? If I go to the Internet, what exactly should I look up?

If you have chemotherapy, you will stay in close contact with your medical oncologist and the chemotherapy nurses. They will be watching carefully to see if you experience side effects from these powerful medicines.

◆ Preparation for Chemotherapy Treatments

One role of chemotherapy in the management of head and neck cancer is to enhance the benefits of radiation therapy. Chemotherapy may also have a *palliative* purpose; that is, to relieve some of the symptoms of cancer without curing it. The medical oncologist is the member of the medical team who specializes in the use of chemotherapy.

Before starting chemotherapy treatments, the medical oncologist will make sure it is safe for you to receive chemotherapy. This is usually done through several blood tests to check the complete blood count (CBC), which includes the hemoglobin, white blood cell count, and platelet count. Other blood tests to study your liver and kidney function will be necessary.

The decision to use chemotherapy is made by your physicians and you. Patients with locally advanced head and neck cancer who undergo radiation therapy are often treated with chemotherapy and radiation during the same time period. There are numerous studies demonstrating the improved benefits of using both radiation and chemotherapy together when treating advanced head and neck cancer.

◆ Chemotherapy Treatments

Once the decision is made to use chemotherapy, the medical oncologist will meet with you to review the chemotherapy drugs and the schedule for administration, the side effects of the therapy, its benefits, and the goals of the therapy. After questions are answered, the medical oncologist will calculate the dose of chemotherapy based on published formulas for the chemotherapy regimens. The exact dosage of chemotherapy is based on the height and weight of the person, results of some of the blood tests that are performed, and the effects the drugs have on other organs of the body.

Because most chemotherapy is given by vein, some medical oncologists and chemotherapy nurses will recommend that a central catheter be placed to administer the chemotherapy. The catheter is called a *peripherally inserted central catheter* (PICC) line. It is a thin, soft, flexible tube that is inserted into a vein in your arm and threaded to a larger vein near your heart. Sometimes a catheter is placed at the chest instead of in the arm. The central catheter can also be used to draw blood samples, administer antibiotics, and administer intravenous fluids or blood products. Some chemotherapy regimens do not require central catheters and can be given by a small catheter placed in a small vein in the back of the hand.

The schedule for chemotherapy can be daily, weekly, or every three weeks depending on the location and type of the cancer and the preference of the medical oncologist. Usually chemotherapy is given in the outpatient chemotherapy unit. There the chemotherapy nurse will again review the chemotherapy regimen and provide important information on how to deal with the side effects of chemotherapy as well as provide contact phone numbers if questions arise. The nurse will recalculate the dose of the chemotherapy and give the orders to a pharmacist who will triple check the prescribed dosage. Depending on the drug, the dose, and the schedule for receiving it, the patient's time in the chemotherapy unit might be as short as 30 minutes or as long as four hours. Some chemotherapy drugs have to be given continuously in a vein for four to five days by a small pump. If this is the case, the nurse will review with you how the pump works and who to call if the pump malfunctions.

◆ Possible Side Effects of Chemotherapy

Some side effects of chemotherapy can include mouth sores, nausea, vomiting, hair loss, numbness of the fingers and toes, hearing loss, kidney damage, and the risk of bleeding and infection. Side effects vary depending on the type of chemotherapy drugs used and the size and frequency of the dose. Usually your medical oncologist will monitor the effects of the chemotherapy with weekly CBC and occasionally blood chemistry tests. If the hemoglobin is too low, you might receive some injections to stimulate the bone marrow to produce more red cells, or a blood transfusion. If the blood platelets count goes too low, some patients will need a platelets transfusion. If the white blood counts go too low and an infection occurs, you may be hospitalized to receive intravenous antibiotics.

Prior to each dose of these cancer-fighting drugs, the chemotherapy nurse or physician will review the side effects of the previous dose and decide if any adjustments need to be made. Most chemotherapy is given concurrently with radiation therapy and, because of this, it is often difficult to determine if a side effect is due to radiation therapy or chemotherapy. Because chemotherapy is an adjunct to radiation therapy, all efforts are made to keep the radiation therapy on schedule. Therefore, if side effects or complications occur, patients may have the chemotherapy modified, delayed, or stopped.

Some patients have cancer in areas of the head and neck that cannot be treated with surgery or radiation therapy, or have cancers that have spread to distant sites such as the bone or lung. In these situations, chemotherapy may be given on a palliative basis. For example, chemotherapy may help to reduce pain, swelling, and shortness of breath, and it may increase appetite. Studies have shown that chemotherapy can improve the quality of life of patients with *metastatic* head and neck cancer, but it has limited impact on increasing overall survival. Questions and concerns about the benefits and goals of chemotherapy should be discussed between the patient and the medical oncologist.

6

Surgery for Cancer of the Larynx

- ◆ **Removal of Small Tumors on the Vocal Folds**
- ◆ **Cordectomy**
- ◆ **Partial Laryngectomy**
- ◆ **Supraglottic Laryngectomy**
- ◆ **Hemilaryngectomy**
- ◆ **Supracricoid Partial Laryngectomy**

- ◆ **Near-Total Laryngectomy**
- ◆ **Total Laryngectomy**
- ◆ **Pharyngo-Laryngo-Esophagectomy**
- ◆ **Neck Dissection**
- ◆ **Complications of Head and Neck Surgery**

As stated in an earlier chapter, surgery is often used as treatment for cancer of the larynx and the surrounding head and neck area. Surgery may be part of a combined treatment before or after either or both radiation therapy and chemotherapy.

The type of surgery for laryngeal cancer is determined by multiple factors including your general health, the size of the tumor, other characteristics of the tumor, and pathologic findings from your biopsy. The surgeon's first objective is to remove the cancer. Following this, the surgeon is concerned that, after surgery, you are able to breathe easily, can swallow foods and liquids safely, and can produce voice and speech. The surgeon will remove only the cancer and leave disease-free tissue undisturbed to function as normally as possible. This is done by having a pathologist examine the removed tissue and ensure that the edges are free of cancer. If necessary, the surgeon may use healthy tissue that is near the area of the cancer to reconstruct structures that were removed. Sometimes the diseased area that must be removed is so large that there is not enough healthy tissue in the surrounding area for this, and tissue from another part of the body must be used for reconstruction. Some structures, such as passageways like the pharynx, can be reconstructed and function quite well. When tumors are very large, vital structures cannot be reconstructed, or they can be only partially reconstructed. The vocal folds and tongue are examples of these. Reconstructions of the vocal folds and tongue do not function as well as the original structures.

This chapter describes some of the surgeries that are performed to remove cancer of the larynx. *These descriptions are very general, and they do not represent every type of surgery for cancer of the larynx.* With modern advances in technology, surgical equipment, and surgical technique, each operation—just like each patient—is different. For example, a procedure may be called a hemilaryngectomy, yet the particulars may be quite different from another surgery that is also considered a form of hemilaryngectomy. Both procedures, and many others, may fit into the overall category of hemilaryngectomy, but the real-life outcomes for breathing, swallowing, and voice for speech can be surprisingly dissimilar. Keep these key points in mind:

- Every cancer and its location is different for every person.
- Every head and neck surgery, even if it has the same name, is different for every person.
- Outcomes from a similar surgery are different for every person.

◆ Removal of Small Tumors on the Vocal Folds

Small superficial (on the surface) tumors are usually removed from the larynx and surrounding areas with a *laser.* This is called endoscopic surgery and is performed "transorally," which means through the mouth. The surgery may also be performed with traditional instruments. Sometimes it is performed at the time of the biopsy and no other treatment is necessary. Endoscopic surgery is most often used for early cancers and has minimal impact on breathing, swallowing, and voice. No reconstruction is necessary. Other than temporary soreness and hoarseness immediately after the surgery, most patients do not have negative long-term effects as a result of this type of procedure. Patients who have endoscopic surgery are usually dismissed from the hospital the same day.

The area of endoscopic laser surgery is one of intensive study and excitement in the field of head and neck cancer surgery. It is a technology and practice that is growing and is now being used for larger and more invasive laryngeal cancers.

◆ Cordectomy

Cordectomy means removal of one vocal cord. Breathing after this surgery is normal. Cordectomy and related surgeries seldom affect swallowing. If swallowing is affected, it is usually for a short time. But the voice will be changed, especially if the entire vocal cord has been removed. The resulting voice usually is breathy and hoarse sounding. It may be softer than before. Speaking loudly may be difficult or impossible. Your voice may improve with time, but your "normal voice" will not return. The surgeon may perform some form of reconstruction at a later date to improve vocal quality.

◆ Partial Laryngectomy

For larger tumors, known as "intermediate" cancers, of certain areas of the larynx, a broad category of surgery called *partial laryngectomy* may be performed. Partial laryngectomy operations, known as "conservation" surgeries, remove the cancerous tissue while preserving three important bodily functions: breathing through the nose and mouth, taking in food and fluids by mouth, and producing a lung-powered voice. This does not mean that everything works as good as new after a conservation surgery. In fact, every type of partial laryngectomy changes swallowing ability or the quality of the voice or both. These changes may be temporary and improve gradually over time. Normal or near-normal swallowing or voice may result. Nevertheless, most partial surgeries cause permanent changes. Changes in breathing seldom are permanent.

Partial laryngectomy means removal of part of the larynx. The cordectomy described above would be considered partial laryngectomy along with other procedures described below. Because the size and location of laryngeal cancers vary from one person to another, there are many types and variations of partial laryngectomy. Some of these surgeries may have the same name or a very similar name, but they can be quite different! This can be very confusing for the patient and family, and it makes it difficult to compare one person's surgery to another person's surgery. As vague as the term *partial laryngectomy* is, it is used in other parts of this book to distinguish it from *near-total laryngectomy* and *total laryngectomy*.

◆ Supraglottic Laryngectomy

In *supraglottic laryngectomy* ("supra-" means "above") the surgeon removes the parts of the larynx above the *true vocal folds,* including the epiglottis and false vocal folds. Immediately after a supraglottic laryngectomy the person breathes through a tube placed in an opening at the front and base of the neck called a tracheostomy. This opening was created in the first stage of the surgery so that breathing remained safe and uninterrupted during the procedure. Tracheostomy is temporary for most people who have supraglottic laryngectomy. The tube is removed and the opening in the neck is allowed to close when the surgeon decides there has been sufficient healing after surgery.

Also during surgery, a small flexible tube, called a *nasogastric (NG) tube*, is placed in the nose, through the esophagus, and into the stomach. This method of receiving liquid food allows the throat to be inactive while it heals from the operation. The NG tube is removed once healing from the surgery has taken place and efforts to swallow are successful.

The epiglottis and false vocal folds removed during supraglottic laryngectomy were part of the valving mechanism that keeps food and liquids from entering the airway during a swallow. Because of this, a person almost always has swallowing difficulties after supraglottic laryngectomy, usually for a month or two, until new swallowing patterns are learned. Frequent coughing, particularly after swallowing, is the main sign that food or liquid has entered the airway. Your speech pathologist may teach you special swallowing techniques that "compensate" for the parts that have been surgically removed. You may practice pulling your tongue back further when swallowing to help shield the true vocal folds and to direct food and liquids toward the esophagus. You may learn other techniques such as holding your breath during a swallow to keep the vocal folds tightly closed. Tucking your chin toward your chest and other changes in head positioning may help to route food and liquids away from the larynx. Some people have longer-term swallowing problems after supraglottic laryngectomy, but most people eventually are able to eat a normal diet.

Because the true vocal folds are not involved in supraglottic laryngectomy, the patient's voice and speech are usually unaffected.

◆ Hemilaryngectomy

Hemilaryngectomy ("hemi" means "half") means removal of half or one side of the larynx. There are many variations of this surgery too. During the operation a tracheostomy tube is placed in an opening in the front and base of the neck for breathing, and a nasogastric tube is put through the nose into the stomach for feeding. These tubes are temporary for most people. After hemilaryngectomy you will have some difficulty with swallowing, at least for a period while you learn ways to compensate for the removal of valves (such as one true vocal cord and one false vocal cord) that previously prevented food from entering the airway. Swallowing liquids is usually the greatest challenge. For most people, these swallowing problems reduce or clear up after a few weeks because the remaining side of the larynx learns to work harder and manages to close the gap left by the tissue that was removed.

The voice is permanently changed after hemilaryngectomy and the result can be quite frustrating. With so much of the vocal mechanism removed, the voice is breathy, rough, lower pitched, and with reduced pitch range. It may tire easily. So much air may escape when the person speaks that attempting to speak loudly or in a noisy environment may be exhausting or impossible. It will be important that you consult your speech pathologist about swallowing and voice concerns.

◆ Supracricoid Partial Laryngectomy

As with other categories of partial laryngectomy, there are many versions of *supracricoid partial laryngectomy*. These procedures are done for advanced cancers. They all have these elements in common: the vocal folds and other parts of the larynx are surgically removed, some of the remaining parts of the larynx are repositioned and may function differently than before, and a permanent tracheostoma for breathing is not necessary.

A person who undergoes a supracricoid partial laryngectomy will awaken from anesthesia with a tracheostomy tube for breathing and a feeding tube for nutrition. These tubes are temporary. After healing has taken place, the person can learn some techniques for swallowing safely without aspirating and should be able to breathe normally and to swallow foods and liquids in a near-normal manner. This may take a while, however. It is not unusual for both a breathing tube and a food tube to remain in place for several weeks.

Although the intelligibility of a person's speech is quite good after supracricoid partial laryngectomy, the quality of the voice is significantly changed. It may be moderately to severely breathy, harsh, or hoarse, and it has limited "tonal" quality. After this surgery, people say it is an effort to produce voice; they must "bear down" to speak, and they cannot speak as many words per breath as they did before. Altogether, these characteristics cause the person to fatigue quickly. A speech pathologist may be able to help the individual speak more efficiently.

◆ Near-Total Laryngectomy

If cancer of the larynx is too extensive to be removed by a partial laryngectomy, but a total laryngectomy is not required, the surgeon may perform a *near-total laryngectomy*. Like other surgeries described previously, several surgical procedures are known as "near-total laryngectomy" or "subtotal laryngectomy." The near-total laryngectomy referred to here means that most of the larynx is removed except a small part of one vocal cord and the main nerve that makes it move. The surgeon uses these remnants of the larynx and other tissue to make a "voice shunt" between the airway and the pharynx (Fig. **6–1**). A person who has had radiation therapy is not a candidate for near-total laryngectomy.

Breathing after near-total laryngectomy is changed dramatically. The opening in the front and center of the lower neck that was created for breathing during the surgery—the tracheostoma—is permanent. The person will always breathe in and out through this opening; air does not move through the mouth and nose because they are no longer connected to the lungs. The person with a near-total laryngectomy usually wears a trach tube or a stoma vent in the tracheostoma until the opening is completely healed and it no longer tends to shrink to a smaller size.

Swallowing after near-total laryngectomy usually becomes normal or close to normal. The nasogastric tube that was placed down the nose at the time of surgery is removed when it is determined that sufficient healing has taken place and the person can start swallowing. The person starts with a diet

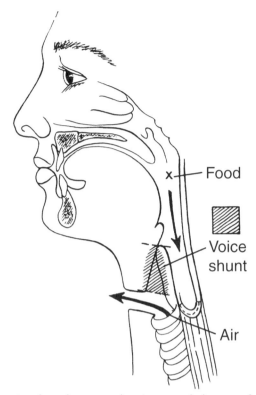

Figure 6–1 The voice shunt between the airway and pharynx after near-total laryngectomy.

of pureed (blenderized) foods and soft foods. The surgeon and speech pathologist are particularly observant of the patient's first attempts to swallow liquids to see if the voice shunt closes completely during swallowing. They will be concerned if there is leakage through the voice shunt and into the trachea when the person swallows. However, slight or occasional leakage is not uncommon. Some people cough when this occurs; others do not. It will be up to your physician, speech pathologist, and you to determine if this leakage causes aspiration (food or liquids going into the lungs) and if it is serious enough to cause additional medical problems. If there is a concern, your speech pathologist will help you experiment with techniques to prevent leakage through the voice shunt when swallowing. (Shine a flashlight into your tracheostoma as you swallow liquids to see if some comes through the voice shunt and starts its way down the trachea). Some patients who experience leakage of fluids through the shunt reduce this by turning their head slightly during the swallow or by tipping the chin toward the chest. Others have succeeded by covering their tracheostoma with a thumb or finger and slightly exhaling (but not enough to produce voice) to help close the voice shunt more tightly.

With just a small part of the larynx remaining and a permanently "rerouted" breathing system, producing voice for speech after near-total

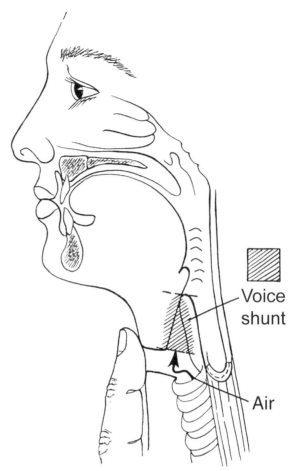

Figure 6–2   Producing voice with the voice shunt after near-total laryngectomy.

laryngectomy will always be different compared with your voice before surgery. Immediately after the operation you will communicate by writing, typing, using gestures, or by pointing to printed words and pictures. See Appendix A for additional suggestions. After some healing has taken place and swelling has reduced, an artificial larynx is used temporarily (see Appendix B).

To produce voice with the voice shunt after adequate healing has occurred, the person must cover the tracheostoma with a thumb or finger and then exhale (Fig. **6–2**). The thumb must be taken away from the stoma to inhale. Eventually, if voice can be produced with effortless, easy *exhalation,* some people are able to wear a valve over the tracheostoma that allows speaking without using a thumb or finger.

The voice shunt will not be ready to produce voice until swelling from the surgery has reduced. This may be as soon as within two or three weeks, but it is more likely to be longer. In fact, it is not unusual for it to take months before the voice shunt works well enough for conversational speech. Most people use an artificial larynx to communicate until the voice shunt produces voice consistently and with little effort. The voice produced by the shunt after near-total laryngectomy usually has a hoarse or strained quality. The voice may sound like it requires considerable effort to produce. This is the case even if producing voice takes little effort.

It will be important for you to consult a speech pathologist experienced in treating patients with near-total laryngectomy so that you can attain the best voice possible and to practice the most natural communication habits with your new voice.

◆ Total Laryngectomy

A *total laryngectomy* means that the entire larynx is removed. A total laryngectomy (also known simply as "*laryngectomy*") is performed when laryngeal cancer is extensive and life threatening. Total laryngectomy can be the first treatment for advanced, aggressive laryngeal cancer. However, total laryngectomy is most often performed when radiation therapy has been administered yet cancer remains, or if there has been a recurrence (return) of cancer when a person has been cancer-free for a period after receiving other treatment in the past. With a total laryngectomy, breathing and voice production are dramatically changed. Swallowing ability changes, but most people report the changes are mild and swallowing improves over time.

Figure **6–3** illustrates the anatomy of the head and neck before laryngectomy. Total laryngectomy includes removal of all the structures and tissues in the area of the thyroid cartilage, also known as the Adam's apple (Fig. **6–4**). After total laryngectomy, there is no pathway for air between the oropharynx (behind the tongue) and the trachea (windpipe). In order for you to continue breathing, the trachea must have direct access to air. For this reason, the surgeon must "reroute" your breathing system and create a permanent opening called a "*stoma*" or "*tracheostoma*" at the front and center of the lower neck. The surgeon brings the trachea to the opening in the neck and sutures the edges together. This opening will range from about the size of a dime coin up to the size of a nickel coin. After the operation, you will breathe through this opening rather than through your nose and mouth. (Refer to Appendix F for additional information.) Because of this, your sense of smell may be reduced, particularly in the early months after your surgery. Your sense of taste may be diminished because most of taste is related to the sense of smell. When you cough, you will have to "catch it" with a tissue or handkerchief at the stoma, not at your nose and mouth. When your nose drips you will not be able to push air through your nose and blow it with any force. Instead, you'll have to wipe away the drips.

Before total laryngectomy, the pharynx is attached to the back of the larynx. When the larynx is removed, the pharynx is left open in the shape of a semicircle facing the front. At this point, the pathway for food between the oropharynx and the esophagus is interrupted. The surgeon will repair the

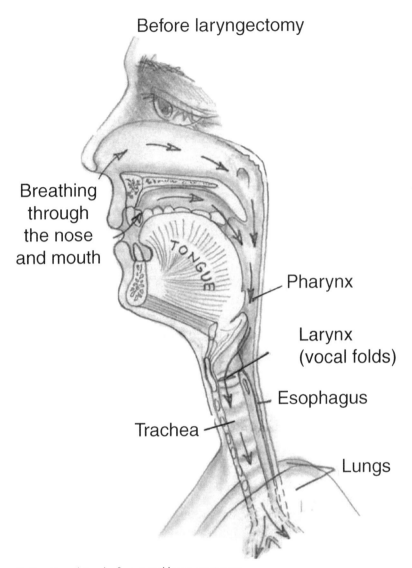

Figure 6–3   Breathing before total laryngectomy.

pharynx by suturing together the remaining edges. After it is sutured, there is a complete pathway for food and there is no way for food or liquids to pass from the esophagus to the trachea.

Total laryngectomy interferes with the muscles that squeeze and move food and liquids down the esophagus and into the stomach. Healing must take place before you can go back to taking food and fluids by mouth. If you eat and drink too soon, food or liquid may lodge where it does not belong, causing problems such as infection and incomplete healing. Usually healing occurs within a week or two of the surgery. The surgeon will give your speech pathologist approval to check your ability to swallow. This test may be an informal

After laryngectomy

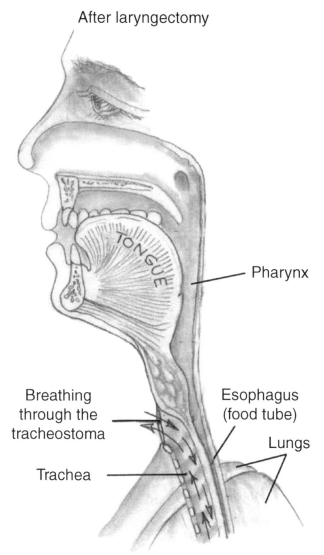

TONGUE

Pharynx

Breathing
through the
tracheostoma

Esophagus
(food tube)

Lungs

Trachea

Figure 6–4 Breathing after total laryngectomy.

one with your speech pathologist or physician observing you while you drink fluids and chew and swallow several different foods. Sometimes an x-ray swallowing test or videofluoroscopic swallow study is performed. This test allows the speech pathologist and physician to observe the entire swallowing mechanism during a moving x-ray to confirm that adequate healing has occurred, to examine how food is moved around in the mouth, to see how quickly food is propelled downward to the stomach, and to observe how long the entire process takes.

Starting out slowly with liquids and soft foods, most people who have had a total laryngectomy are able to return to their normal diet within a month after surgery. Some laryngectomized people (also known as "*laryngectomees*") say they must chew food more thoroughly before swallowing, and it takes longer to eat a meal. They may need to swallow "harder" to give the food a bigger push down into the esophagus. Others say they must drink more fluids with their meals to help move food down toward the stomach. For some laryngectomized people, the opening into the esophagus is narrower than before and it doesn't seem to "stretch" as much. For them, swallowing may be difficult and slow, and some types of food must be avoided altogether. For a small percentage of laryngectomized people, the diet must be made up of liquids and blenderized foods only. These problems usually result from surgery for disease in later stages that require more extensive removal of tissue combined with either or both radiation therapy and chemotherapy. For more information about nutrition and swallowing after total laryngectomy, see Appendix D.

Immediately after total laryngectomy the person will need to communicate by using the nurse's call light or a bell or sound maker, clapping hands, writing, typing, using gestures, and pointing to printed words and pictures. At home, these same methods may be used, including using e-mail instead of the telephone. See Appendix A for a listing of methods of communicating after head and neck cancer treatments.

With the entire larynx removed, producing voice for speech will be completely different. When you are ready your speech pathologist will help you use an artificial larynx. How can you determine when you are ready? You are ready when (1) you are interested in trying an artificial larynx; (2) you have reduced swelling in your face, mouth, and neck; (3) you are swallowing your saliva; and (4) you do not have pain when you make speech movements with your tongue, lips, and jaw. See Appendix B for more information on artificial larynges.

Two other methods of speech after total laryngectomy—*tracheoesophageal puncture* (TEP) and esophageal speech—are also described in Appendix B.

◆ Pharyngo-Laryngo-Esophagectomy

Pharyngo-laryngo-esophagectomy (also spelled as one long word without hyphens) is a very complex surgery to remove cancer that invades deeply into the pharynx (throat), larynx (vocal folds), and esophagus (food passage to the stomach). The operation removes all of these structures.

Reconstruction of the larynx is not a possibility, but it is possible to reconstruct the pharynx and esophagus to make a new passage for swallowing food and liquids. This requires taking tissue from other areas of the body. Surgeons use different methods of reconstruction based on their preference and what other tissue works best. Skin from the chest, called a *pectoral myocutaneous flap*, may be rolled into a tube to substitute as part of the pharynx. Similarly, skin from the forearm, called a radial *forearm free flap*, can be rolled and sewn in to replace the entire pharynx. Another possibility is to use a part of the small intestine called the *jejunum* as a replacement for the pharynx. If the surgeon must remove the larynx, pharynx, and most or all of the esophagus, a procedure called *gastric pull-up* or gastric interposition may be performed. The stomach is actually pulled up and sutured to the throat.

These are very simplified descriptions of very complex operations. Surgeons from other specialty areas often participate in these procedures, such as when removal of pharyngeal, laryngeal, and esophageal cancer requires reconstruction of the passage for swallowing by moving tissue from the chest, arm, or abdomen, or if it involves pulling up the stomach to serve as part of the throat. Again, and unfortunately, when the larynx is completely removed, it cannot be reconstructed.

Breathing after pharyngo-laryngo-esophagectomy is similar to that after near-total laryngectomy and total laryngectomy. Because the entire larynx is removed, the patient will always breathe through a permanent tracheostoma at the front and base of the neck. Changes in breathing after pharyngo-laryngo-esophagectomy are similar to those shown in Fig. **6–4** after total laryngectomy; however, the reconstruction of the food passage after pharyngo-laryngo-esophagectomy is not shown in this figure.

Swallowing ability changes after these surgeries. The back of the tongue and any remaining original muscles at the back of the throat must "work harder" to propel food and liquid back and down into the reconstructed swallowing tube. Unlike the original pharynx and esophagus, the new swallowing tube does little or nothing to help food and liquids proceed on their way toward the stomach. As a result, each swallow may take longer. Many patients report that they must chew their food more thoroughly, take smaller bites, eat less hard and chunky foods, drink more liquids during a meal, and allow more time for each meal. For some patients, the reconstructed swallowing tube gradually tightens and becomes narrow, particularly where it has been sewn to other structures. When this occurs, a physician may need to dilate or stretch the tube to allow foods and liquids to pass through it faster and with less effort.

For most patients after pharyngo-laryngo-esophagectomy, there are two possible methods of speaking. The first is using an artificial larynx. The second method is tracheoesophageal puncture (TEP) with a voice prosthesis (see Appendix B). Note that, usually, the "puncture" process after pharyngo-laryngo-esophagectomy is referred to as a tracheoesophageal puncture or TEP, even though the esophagus has been removed and reconstructed with tissue from another part of the body. Similarly, speech produced after this procedure is usually called tracheoesophageal speech, or TEP speech.

For several reasons the surgeon may postpone performing a TEP after pharyngo-laryngo-esophagectomy longer than after a total laryngectomy. This decision is usually based on the surgeon wanting the patient to be well healed from that major surgery, adjusted to changes in swallowing ability, and recovered from any radiation therapy or chemotherapy treatments.

◆ Neck Dissection

If the tumor has spread or is at risk to spread from the larynx to the lymph nodes in the neck, an operation called a "complete neck dissection" or "modified neck dissection" will be performed, usually at the same time as the surgery involving the larynx.

A *neck dissection* is the surgical removal of the lymph nodes and possibly vessels, nerves, and muscles on one or both sides of the neck. When cancer of the larynx spreads, it usually goes to the tissues in the neck first, rather than to distant parts of the body. This is why, if there is any evidence that the cancer may have begun to spread, it is important to remove the tissues that are most likely to contain tumor cells. Adding a neck dissection to laryngeal surgery does not significantly increase the risks of the operation, and it can improve the chance of eliminating disease. Neck dissections are usually done for supraglottic cancers and advanced *glottic cancers.*

The muscle and tissue removed during neck dissection may cause changes in appearance, sensation, and function. When sufficient healing has occurred, the sutures are removed. After swelling from surgery has gone down, your neck may be thinner than before—your shirt collar size will be smaller. A complete neck dissection will cause the skin on the neck, and sometimes the face and ear on that side, to be numb because sensory nerves had to be cut or stretched to remove the cancer during the surgery. Over time, people usually experience tingling or a prickling sensation at the neck and face, and they notice that some feeling gradually returns to those areas.

For many people, a neck dissection causes some reduction in the range of movement of the neck, especially when combined with radiation therapy. But it usually does not prevent them from turning their head or raising and lowering it. Also, if the shoulder nerve has been removed or stretched, the shoulder may appear "dropped" and it may take more effort to raise the arm up. The shoulder may tire more easily on the side where the neck dissection was performed. Some people report activities that require them to raise their arm, such as combing their hair or reaching up to a high shelf, are difficult. Your golf swing may change after neck dissection. Carrying a toolbox or handbag or lifting anything heavier than a pound or two on the affected side may be uncomfortable. See Appendix G for more information and exercises for improving posture and head, neck, shoulder, and arm mobility. Ask your physician if these are appropriate for you.

Neck dissection does not have a direct effect on speaking or swallowing. If you have a neck dissection on one side or on both sides along with a total laryngectomy, use of a neck-type artificial larynx may need to be postponed until swelling has reduced at the neck. However, use of an oral-type artificial larynx may be a possibility as soon as within a few days or a week after surgery.

◆ Complications of Head and Neck Surgery

Every operation, including those for head and neck cancer, involves certain risks and potential complications. However, for most patients, the possibility of having any of these complications is not high. Remember, before surgery a thorough physical examination will help identify conditions that could cause complications during or after surgery. This examination, together with your medical history and a review of the medications you take, helps your physicians determine your candidacy for surgery. If your physicians have particular concerns, they will discuss them with you. If you have any particular concerns, bring them up for discussion with your physicians.

One complication after surgery is called a *fistula*. A fistula is a small opening along or near the incision line that creates a passageway from one area to another, for example, an opening between the pharynx and the skin of the neck. In this case, mucus drains from the pharynx through the fistula and prevents the incision from healing properly. A fistula can delay the total healing process.

Fistulas occur more frequently after surgery in people who have had radiation therapy before surgery. The radiation weakens the tissues, which then break down more easily, and healing is compromised. Although not much can be done to speed up the healing of a fistula, it usually heals by itself in a few weeks. If you develop a fistula, you may help it heal by keeping the area clean and changing the bandages or absorbent packing frequently. Your physician or nurse will show you how to do this and advise how often to do it. You may have to be fed by a tube until the fistula heals completely.

7

Surgery for Cancer of the Tongue

- ◆ Types of Surgery
- ◆ Breathing during and after Tongue Surgery
- ◆ The Tongue and Swallowing
- ◆ The Tongue and Speech Production
- ◆ Radiation Therapy and Chemotherapy
- ◆ Use of a Palatal Augmentation Prosthesis after Surgery on the Tongue
- ◆ Speech and Swallowing after Total Glossectomy and Total Laryngectomy

Cancer of the tongue can occur by itself. Tumor growth can involve other parts of the mouth, however, such as the lips, gums, the floor of the mouth, the jaw (mandible), the roof of the mouth (palate), the tonsils, and the larynx. Even a small tumor in the tongue can make it stiff, slow, "clumsy," and less able to manipulate food for easy, normal swallowing. The same tumor may make it difficult for the tongue to perform the precise and very rapid movements required for normal speech.

This section presents descriptions of some surgeries to remove cancer of the tongue. *These descriptions are very general, and they do not represent every type of surgery for cancer of the tongue or other parts of the mouth.*

Some names of surgical procedures for cancer of the tongue may lead to confusion. For example, a procedure may be called "hemiglossectomy," yet the particulars may be quite different from another surgery that is also considered a form of hemiglossectomy. Both procedures, and many others, may fit into the overall category of hemiglossectomy, but the real-life outcomes for speech, swallowing, and sometimes breathing can be surprisingly different. Keep these key points in mind:

- Every cancer and its location is different for every person.
- Every surgery for cancer of the tongue or other parts of the mouth, even if it has the same name as another, is different for every person.
- Outcomes from a similar surgery are different for every person.

◆ Types of Surgery

Surgery may be necessary to remove a cancerous tumor of the tongue. Surgery may be preceded or followed by either or both radiation therapy and chemotherapy (Chapters 4 and 5). Some tumors on the tongue can be surgically removed using *electrocautery* or a laser, and recovery afterward is rapid. Removal of small tumors, depending on their location, may cause little if any change in speech or swallowing after healing has taken place. Removal of larger tumors may cause significant speech and swallowing problems.

Two common medical terms for the surgical removal of the tongue are *partial glossectomy* and *total glossectomy*. The term partial glossectomy is vague. Removal of a small part of the tongue can be referred to as a partial glossectomy (Fig. **7–1**). Yet that same term can refer to removal of up to 50% of the tongue. *Hemiglossectomy,* a form of partial glossectomy, means removal of ~50% of the anterior tongue, and it often means removal of all or most of one side of the tongue (Fig. **7–2**). Subtotal glossectomy means 50 to 75% of the tongue is surgically removed. "Total glossectomy" is a rare operation. It refers to removal of the entire tongue, but it also may be the term used when more than 75% of the tongue is removed. After total glossectomy the tongue

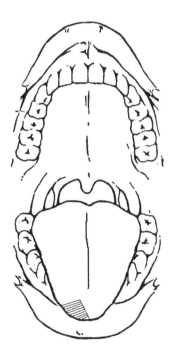

Figure 7–1   An example of partial glossectomy.

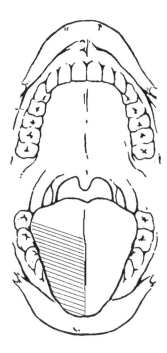

Figure 7–2   An example of hemiglossectomy.

remnant is insufficient to enable near-normal swallowing or speech. "Reconstruction" of the tongue may take place to fill in the space left when a major portion of the tongue is removed. In this case, the surgeon and/or a head and neck reconstructive surgeon will "transfer" tissue from another part of the body, such as from the forearm or chest. This tissue—muscle and skin with blood vessels—is called a *free flap*. The remaining tongue may be able to move this tissue sufficiently to aid in moving some foods and liquids to the back of the throat for swallowing, as well as to make some speech sounds. The free flap does not have the capability of moving on its own, nor does it have the sense of taste or full sensation.

If your surgeon or medical team is recommending surgery for cancer of the tongue, ask them to describe the part of the tongue that must be removed and request that they refer to Fig. **7–3** to draw in that area. If there will be reconstruction of the tongue with tissue from another part of your body, ask for details. Again, the treatment is individualized for each patient and situation and may be quite variable.

◆ Breathing during and after Tongue Surgery

When about half or more of the tongue must be removed, the surgeon usually performs a tracheostomy and places a breathing tube at the front and center of the base of the neck. This is necessary because surgery on the tongue causes

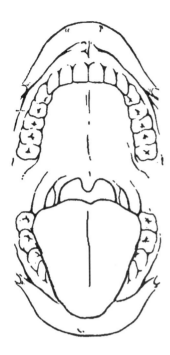

Figure 7–3 If surgery is recommended for cancer of the tongue, ask your physician to draw in the area that must be removed.

it to swell, making normal breathing difficult. The tracheostomy allows the person to breathe safely and easily during and after the surgery. The remaining tissue is swollen. As swelling reduces and breathing becomes unobstructed, the trach tube can be removed and the opening in the neck will close. Ask your surgeon about this.

In rare cases when a partial or total glossectomy is performed together with a near-total or total laryngectomy, the tracheostomy will be permanent. To learn more about permanent tracheostomy, see Appendix F. For more information on near-total laryngectomy or total laryngectomy, see Chapter 6 and Appendix B.

◆ The Tongue and Swallowing

Immediately after surgery you may not be able to swallow until healing takes place and swelling reduces. For some people, a nasogastric (NG) feeding tube is necessary for a period of time. Will surgery on your tongue permanently affect your ability to swallow? For some people there are no permanent changes; for others, the changes are significant and permanent. *It depends on what part of the tongue is removed and how much of it is removed.* Some people eventually eat a normal diet, though eating a meal may continue to take longer. Smaller bites and more chewing may be required. After the resection of advanced cancers, other people may be able to swallow only pureed/blenderized foods. Some may require special utensils that place food or liquid further back in the mouth and closer to the pharynx (back of the throat). A lesser number may be unable to take a sufficient amount of food and liquid by mouth and must depend on a *percutaneous endoscopic gastrostomy* (PEG) tube as a route for some or all of their nutrition (Appendix C). It will be important to see a speech pathologist for assistance with swallowing. For information about swallowing, see Chapter 2 and Appendix D.

◆ The Tongue and Speech Production

The tongue is made up of muscles that produce movements and sounds for speech. When part of the tongue is removed, speech often changes. How much does it change? *Again, it depends on what part of the tongue is removed and how much of it is removed.* The more tongue removed, the greater the speech impairment. Effects on speech can range from normal speech if the cancer is not at the tip of the tongue and the cancer is removed when it is quite small, to only slightly distorted speech that others have no difficulty understanding, to no usable speech at all. Consultation with a speech pathologist knowledgeable about these conditions is helpful and important for rehabilitation. The speech pathologist may recommend exercises for you to utilize and preserve as much movement of the remaining tongue as possible. Speech therapy often focuses on making sounds that are as similar as possible to the ones you can no longer make due to reduced tissue and movement of the tongue in the mouth. You may learn to make substitute or "compensatory" movements with the lips, cheeks, and jaw in combination with the teeth to make sounds as similar as possible to speech sounds you can no longer make in the customary manner. Other changes may make speech more *intelligible,* such as speaking more slowly, exaggerating vocal and inflection patterns, and using gestures and pantomimes that are easily recognizable. If you have had surgery on your tongue and your speech has been affected, practice the "Six Tips for Better Communication after Treatments for Cancer of the Larynx or Tongue" in Appendix I.

◆ Radiation Therapy and Chemotherapy

Radiation therapy with or without chemotherapy may be a part of treatment for tongue cancer. During these treatments and for some time afterward, the tongue and entire mouth and throat may become swollen, sore, and dry, making swallowing extremely difficult (see Chapters 4 and 5). Under these conditions, feeding by tube—usually a PEG—is often necessary to receive nutrition until the person can take adequate food and fluids by mouth (see Appendix C).

As described earlier, radiation therapy causes fibrosis. This means the tongue becomes less mobile, which leads to additional swallowing and speech problems. A speech pathologist may recommend tongue exercises for you to carry out throughout the day to minimize this stiffening and to help the tongue maintain flexibility. Range of motion and flexibility are very important for the tongue to "reach" particular locations in the mouth and to move quickly and in a coordinated way for both swallowing and speech. Ask your speech pathologist if exercises for the tongue are right for you, and if so, to review with you the tongue exercises described in Appendix E.

◆ Use of a Palatal Augmentation Prosthesis after Surgery on the Tongue

Another way to improve speech and swallowing after much or most of the tongue has been surgically removed is to lower the roof of the mouth. The roof of the mouth is also known as the palate. When the palate is lowered, it is easier for the remaining or reconstructed tongue to come into contact with it. This may aid in preparing and moving foods and liquids around in the mouth before swallowing. Additionally, a lowered palate may provide a hard surface that is "within reach" for the reduced tongue to press up against for the production of speech sounds. The maxillofacial prosthodontist, a dentist who specializes in dental and facial restoration and reconstruction, is the member of the health care team who constructs a device known as a *palatal augmentation prosthesis*. The prosthesis must be custom-made for each patient. It may be attached to the teeth and fits snugly up against the roof of the mouth. The process for being fitted for a palatal augmentation prosthesis may require special imaging tests and impressions of the patient's unique oral cavity to determine the best configuration of the prosthesis.

◆ Speech and Swallowing after Total Glossectomy and Total Laryngectomy

Sometimes cancer extends beyond the tongue and includes the larynx, or *voice box*. When cancer of the tongue is combined with cancer of the larynx, the seriousness of the disease is compounded and the debilitating, life-changing consequences of the disease and its treatment are greater. In these cases, to save the life of the person, the treatment most likely to be recommended is the removal of part or all of the tongue and larynx. If you have cancer of the tongue and larynx, the disease and treatments for it will cause permanent changes in swallowing and speech and usually in breathing.

When most or all of the tongue is removed as well as the entire larynx, the person may be able to produce some speech with a tracheoesophageal puncture voice (see Appendix B). The resulting speech is not normal and some persons find the quality and intelligibility of their speech after these extensive surgical changes too "different" to be acceptable. Glossectomized-laryngec-tomized persons will very frequently find themselves in communication situations in which their speech is not understood. They may need to use other methods of communication. Some of the methods described in Appendix A are possibilities.

8

In the Hospital after Surgery for Cancer of the Larynx

- ◆ How Long Will I Be in the Hospital?
- ◆ What Is All This Equipment?
- ◆ Tracheostomy for Breathing
- ◆ Tracheostomy Tube
- ◆ Oxygen
- ◆ Intravenous Fluids
- ◆ Nasogastric Feeding Tube
- ◆ Drainage
- ◆ Pain

◆ How Long Will I Be in the Hospital?

This is one of the first questions people ask when they learn they will have surgery. Your surgeon will answer that question. It depends on the type and extent of your surgery, your general condition, your surgeon's preference, and the standard practice of the hospital. After surgery for smaller, superficial tumors, you may be released the same day as the surgery. After surgery for more extensive tumors, you will be taken to a recovery area and then to a hospital room.

◆ What Is All This Equipment?

Some equipment may be in place after you have laryngeal surgery. For various partial laryngectomy surgeries, you may become aware of bandages, tubes, an intravenous fluid line, and possibly a nasogastric feeding tube. You may have a tracheostomy tube at your neck for breathing, an oxygen tube, and possibly drain tubes attached to your body (Fig. **8–1**). After near-total laryngectomy and total laryngectomy, all of these will be in place. Again, depending on the kind of surgery, your face and neck may be quite swollen. Neither you nor your family should become worried about this or at the sight of the equipment. It is all part of routine procedure designed to help you recover quickly from surgery. If you have sponge pads and bandages at your neck, for example, they are there only temporarily to absorb fluids and protect the incision until it begins to heal. If you have a tracheostomy at the base of your neck (your surgeon will discuss this with you before the surgery), you may be receiving free-flowing oxygen there for easy breathing.

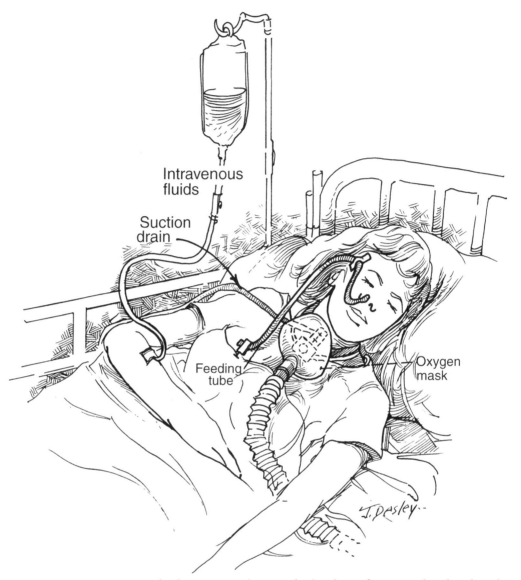

Figure 8–1 Medical equipment that *may* be in place after some head and neck surgeries. Ask your physician what equipment will be necessary if you have surgery.

◆ Tracheostomy for Breathing

At the beginning of many surgeries for cancer of the larynx, after you are anesthetized, the surgeon must make an opening at the base of the neck to allow you to breathe easily, safely, and without aspiration and without interruption during surgery. The surgery to make the opening is called a tracheotomy. The opening in the neck is called a *tracheostomy*. It may be temporary or permanent, depending on how much of the larynx must be removed. Usually the tracheostomy is permanent only for near-total laryngectomy and total laryngectomy. Ask your surgeon if you will need a tracheostomy and if it will be temporary or permanent.

For some surgeries such as cordectomy, partial laryngectomy, supraglottic laryngectomy, *transoral laser surgeries,* and variations of these that leave some of the larynx intact, the surgeon does not disconnect the airway from the food passage. The tracheostomy is usually temporary until laryngeal tissues have healed and they can resume their function.

After extensive surgeries such as near-total laryngectomy and total laryngectomy and variations of these, in which most or all of the larynx is removed, the surgeon completely disconnects the airway from the food passage. The tracheostomy will be permanent because all protective tissues and functions of the larynx are removed. Whether the tracheostomy is temporary or permanent, for a period after your surgery you may need to wear a tracheostomy tube in the opening at the neck to keep it open.

◆ Tracheostomy Tube

Tracheostomy tubes or *trach tubes* are made of metal or a type of a plastic material. There are many types of trach tubes. Typically they are placed in the opening at the base of your neck to hold it open during the operation and immediately after it.

If you have a temporary tracheostomy, a trach tube may need to be in the opening until you can breathe adequately through the nose and mouth, and you can swallow without food and liquid going to your lungs. For those with a permanent tracheostomy, the tube will hold the stoma open until it heals and stays open on its own. For more information about living with a permanent tracheostomy, see Appendix F.

The metal trach tube illustrated in Fig. **8–2** consists of three parts: an outer tube called the "outer cannula," an inner tube called the "inner cannula," and a small device called the "introducer" (also known as an "obturator"). The outer tube holds the stoma open. It is taken out of the stoma occasionally to be cleaned, perhaps in the morning and in the evening. You will be instructed on how to do this and how often by a caregiver, perhaps an ear, nose, and throat (ENT) nurse.

The introducer is a smooth-tipped instrument that fits into the outer cannula of the tracheostomy tube. By using the introducer, you will be able to insert the tracheostomy tube easily into the stoma. Once the tube is in, the introducer is removed. The inner cannula fits tightly into the outer tube, but it can be removed easily. The inner cannula should be taken out and cleaned frequently. When the trach tube is in the stoma, it is held in place by a padded

Metal trach tube

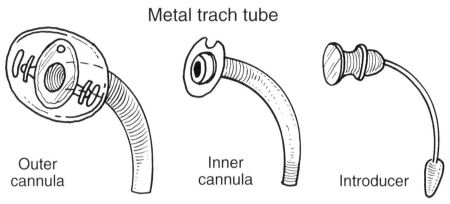

Outer cannula   Inner cannula   Introducer

Figure 8–2   Parts of a metal trach tube. Ask your physician if you will need a trach tube.

neckband and Velcro strips or "tie tapes," which are attached to the sides of the outer cannula and go around your neck and fasten in the back.

When you wake up from surgery, you will see that the tracheostomy tube has already been inserted. If your tracheostomy is temporary, your physician will eventually want it to close when you are breathing and swallowing adequately. He or she will discuss with you when the trach tube may be removed. Usually, after the trach tube is removed, a bandage may be placed over the location of the opening while it is healing, and the opening closes on its own.

If you have a permanent tracheostomy, the purpose of the tracheostomy tube is to help the stoma heal properly, and you will probably be wearing it when you leave the hospital. Eventually, most people with permanent tracheostomies find that, in time, they no longer need the tube to keep the stoma open because the stoma stays open on its own. Instead of a plastic or metal tracheostomy tube, you may eventually wear a short tube called a stoma vent, button, or stud made of soft silicone. Because each patient responds a little differently to treatment, however, *you should leave the trach tube out only upon the advice of your physician.* Otherwise, the stoma may shrink too much and you may have difficulty breathing. If this occurs, seek medical attention at once. Again, you will receive instructions, probably from a nurse, on the home care of the tracheostomy tube.

After laryngeal surgery, the lungs and trachea often secrete a great deal of mucus, at least for the first few days. There are two ways to get rid of these secretions if you have a tracheostomy. Either you will expel it through the tracheostomy tube by coughing, or the nurse may place a "suction tube" into the tracheostomy tube and apply gentle suction to remove the secretions. When suction is used to remove secretions, it may cause you to cough; this usually is beneficial because it will help clear out the mucus. It often takes a while before you remember to hold a tissue or handkerchief at the opening in the neck when you cough rather than to hold it at the mouth.

◆ Oxygen

Often after head and neck surgery the patient receives oxygen to make breathing easy. If the surgery does not require a tracheostomy, the oxygen will be delivered at the nose or the mouth. If a tracheostomy is performed, the oxygen will be delivered through a tube into a mask or collar at the neck. The oxygen is humidified and helps moisten the air passing into the lungs. This is not the same as a ventilator or respirator that pushes air into the lungs when a person cannot breathe independently. The free-flowing oxygen with moisture substitutes for the humidifying function that was provided by the nose and mouth before the surgery and tracheostomy.

◆ Intravenous Fluids

If you have had surgery on your tongue, throat, or larynx, you probably won't be given anything to eat or drink immediately after surgery. There are two main reasons for this. First, the tissues of the throat and surrounding areas must be protected to begin healing, and second, your digestive system isn't ready for food immediately after surgery. When you are anesthetized, your digestive system goes to sleep with the rest of your body. Just as it may take a few days for you to stop feeling groggy, it may take some time for your digestive system to resume functioning normally. You may receive intravenous (IV) fluids.

For intravenous fluids, a needle is inserted into a vein. The needle is attached to a line (tube) through which fluids will pass. These fluids will provide calories and electrolytes (sodium, potassium, chloride, and phosphorus). Their purpose is to keep you well hydrated. You may gradually begin receiving liquid food as well as any medication you need through a separate tube known as a nasogastric (NG) feeding tube. Intravenous fluids may be stopped as you increase to the full amount of liquid food through the feeding tube.

◆ Nasogastric Feeding Tube

As described in previous chapters of this book, when the pharynx and related areas are surgically cut and then sutured closed, the sutures must not be irritated or subjected to stress or pressure to heal properly. This means that you should not swallow foods or liquids immediately afterward. That is why, when you are still anesthetized, a small soft flexible tube called a nasogastric (NG) tube is passed from your nose through the pharynx and down the esophagus and into your stomach. The tube is usually taped to your nose, neck, or forehead. When the digestive system is ready, all the liquid food and fluids necessary for adequate nutrition, as well as medicine, can pass through the tube while the pharynx is healing. Receiving food through a tube is called enteral feeding. During and after NG tube feedings, patients sometimes have a feeling of "heartburn" while this tube is in place. This disappears shortly after the tube is removed. For more information on NG tube feeding, see Appendix C.

The NG feeding tube is usually removed by the physician within a few weeks after the head and neck surgery, depending on the surgery. After removal of the tube, you may be advised to swallow only liquids, pureed (blenderized) foods, or soft foods—the foods that can be swallowed without aspiration and those that "go down" easily for you. More information on swallowing after various laryngeal or tongue surgeries can be found under the headings of particular types of surgery in Chapters 6 and 7 and Appendix D.

There are exceptions to having a feeding tube placed down the nose. If you have a total laryngectomy with tracheoesophageal puncture, the feeding tube may be passed through the puncture opening rather than down the nose. With this route, the feeding tube goes through the tracheostoma, through the back wall of the trachea and through the front wall of the esophagus, then down the esophagus and into the stomach. Removal of this tube usually follows the same schedule as for an NG tube. For information about total laryngectomy and tracheoesophageal puncture, see Chapter 6 and Appendix B.

For various medical reasons some patients may require prolonged tube feeding. In these cases, a different route for nutrition than a nasogastric tube may be necessary. An example of this would be for receiving nutrition after surgery and during radiation therapy when the entire head and neck area may be too irritated to tolerate the NG tube in the throat. The most common feeding tube of this type is called a percutaneous endoscopic gastrostomy (PEG) tube (see Appendix C). A PEG is a flexible tube that is inserted through the abdomen into the stomach. If necessary, an extension of this tube may be placed into the small bowel. These feeding tubes provide the same essentials as the NG tube: water, nutrition, and medications. With a PEG, the only part of the tube you see is the disk on your abdomen connected to a short flexible tube where liquid food is administered.

◆ Drainage

After some head and neck surgeries, the field of surgery under the skin incision may produce excessive serum and tissue fluid for several days after the surgery. These fluids are removed by one or more suction drain tubes. By removing these secretions from under the incision, the healing process is faster and healthier with less scarring. Usually within a few days after surgery the amount of daily serum and tissue fluid secretion has decreased enough that you will no longer need the drainage apparatus.

◆ Pain

Although most patients who have had extensive laryngeal surgery do experience some pain after the operation, many are surprised to discover that the pain is less than that associated with other surgeries. If you have pain, however, let your physician and nurses know. Pain medication will be available if you need it. Everyone wants you to be as comfortable as possible while you're recovering from surgery.

9

Coping during and after Cancer Treatments

It is natural for a person to become anxious, worried, and sad when faced with cancer and treatments for it. These feelings may occur soon after the diagnosis, before and during treatments, during a hospital stay, after returning home—or just about any time. They are common, normal, and predictable feelings. Your appearance may have changed. You may feel disfigured. What was simple and automatic—breathing, swallowing, and speaking—may now require you to learn new behaviors and make big adjustments. You may feel the changes in your life are monumental and overwhelming. You may become depressed.

People have different ways of dealing with feelings of loss, sadness, and depression. Some people say their spirits are lifted by being with friends or relatives. Other people say they overcome their feelings of depression by visiting their place of worship, reading uplifting material, returning to work or volunteering, taking short trips, or meeting other cancer survivors who have "been there." Some people find that when they concentrate their efforts on improving any swallowing or speaking difficulty they now have, their depression gradually reduces.

If you have difficulty overcoming feelings of depression, do not hesitate to speak with your physician about it. He or she may prescribe an antidepressant or other medication that may relieve intense feelings of sadness and other symptoms of depression. Remember that seeking help for depression is part of "taking charge" and moving forward. Additionally your physician may refer you to a counselor, such as a psychiatrist, psychologist, hospital chaplain, or other therapist skilled in helping people adjust to difficult, sad, and frightening situations.

If you have had a total laryngectomy, your speech pathologist may introduce you to another person who has recovered from a surgery similar to yours, or refer you to a New Voice Club or to the International Association of Laryngectomees (see Chapter 10 and Appendix H). Several services, support groups, and organizations are available in most cities and some towns. A social worker may help you locate a support group. Even if you do not usually participate in support organizations, you may find that meeting and mingling with people in similar circumstances can help you move forward constructively, get back into the mainstream of life, and view the present and your future more positively. Spouses of people with cancer often appreciate the advice and support from other spouses who have been through similar experiences.

You will need determination to adjust to changes in swallowing, voice, and speech. You are not completely alone in this adjustment. Most people find that their family and friends are going through changes too. Usually they are very concerned and ready to help in some way. From the beginning, be as clear and open as possible with the people who are close to you. Explain what changes have occurred due to surgery or other treatments and how you are learning to do some of the "basics" all over again. Tell them you had cancer and where it was located, and describe the treatments you have experienced. *Also, it is important that others understand that cancer is not contagious.* Scientific evidence indicates that cancer is no more contagious than a heart attack or a broken leg.

Do not overlook other ways to cope—ways to focus your efforts on living more fully as you confront a serious illness. Consider exercise, relaxation, meditation, spirituality, yoga, humor, music, art, writing in a journal, and spending time with pets.

◆ Cancer Survivorship: How to Cope and Thrive after Treatment

In many ways, surviving cancer is a process. It begins the moment cancer enters your life and continues during and well after your treatment. People sometimes use the term *survivor* to describe anyone who is still alive after having received a diagnosis of cancer. But they also might use it to describe someone with no evidence of active disease after treatment.

Though you're deservedly relieved that you've won cancer's major physical battle, the end of treatment may also mean facing many new challenges and concerns. Recovery may require a different way of thinking about yourself and relating to others. Here are some suggestions to help you make the transition from patient to survivor.

Follow-up Care Can Reduce Worry

After cancer treatment, you may worry about the possible return of cancer. But being aware of important changes in your health such as trouble eating, new lumps or bumps, and new, unexplained and persistent pain, in addition to getting regular follow-up medical care, may help alleviate some of these concerns.

During follow-up care appointments, your physician will usually evaluate your medical history and examine you for evidence of recurrence of cancer, the development of other cancers, and side effects from cancer treatment. Depending on the type of cancer and treatment you've had, your physician may also do other tests. These might include blood tests or imaging studies, such as x-rays and scans. In some instances, physical or occupational therapy may help enhance recovery.

Tips for Managing Your Follow-up Medical Care

- Ask your cancer specialist how frequently you should have checkups, what your checkups should involve, and what changes in your health might indicate a problem. The answers to these questions depend on the type and stage of cancer you had and on your general health. No two people have exactly the same tests or follow-up care. For example, someone treated for an aggressive cancer might be seen more regularly than someone with a less-aggressive cancer.
- Be aware of changes in your health especially those that your physician has indicated might reveal potential problems, and tell your physician if these occur.
- Choose a physician you're comfortable with to handle your follow-up care, if you have a choice. This may be your primary care physician or one of the specialists who treated your cancer.
- Check with your insurance provider to see whether coverage of follow-up care is subject to any restrictions. If it is, find out if your state provides health insurance for people who are more difficult to insure. Or look into group insurance options through professional, fraternal, or political organizations.
- Keep detailed records of your cancer diagnosis, treatment, complications, and contact information for your physicians. Use the records checklist in Chapter 3 to help get you started.

Taking Care of Your Body after Treatment

After your cancer treatment is complete, focus on healthy habits, such as eating well and exercising regularly, 30 to 60 minutes on most days of the week, when appropriate. Depending on the type of cancer and treatment you've had and how well your body tolerates its treatment, you may experience aftereffects for months or years. You may wonder what aftereffects are normal and what signs and symptoms suggest that your cancer might have returned. Here are some effects commonly noted following cancer treatment and some tips for coping with them.

- *Pain:* Pain related to cancer may stem from several factors. The cancer itself can cause pain by destroying tissue around the area in which it was located. Surgery can also cause pain, as can radiation, which may result in burning sensations or scars. And chemotherapy can have many potentially painful side effects, including mouth sores and nerve damage. Your physician may prescribe medications, physical therapy, or techniques such as nerve blocks or surgery. Relaxation techniques such as deep breathing or meditation or massage may help you control pain on your own. As a general rule, pain caused by cancer doesn't go away and isn't intermittent. If your pain goes away on its own within a few days, it's probably not due to cancer. Report pain to your physician if it's a severe or persistent problem.

- *Fatigue:* During cancer treatment, fatigue can occur for many reasons, including poor nutrition or depression. Fatigue may also be brought on by the disease itself or may be a side effect of treatment. Most fatigue that follows cancer treatment eventually subsides, but it may take months. Although you may not know the cause of fatigue that follows cancer treatment, you can keep your fatigue in check. Try to plan your activities for times when you usually have the most energy. Relaxation techniques such as meditation or yoga may help. Your physician also may suggest changes in your diet or exercise routines.

- *Changes in your sex life:* Your sex life may be affected in several ways, both physically and emotionally. Your interest in sex may diminish, or you may have problems with sexual function such as impotence or painful intercourse. You may become infertile. Talking with your partner and trying a different approach to sex may help. Most importantly, tell your physician if these things are happening. He or she may have medical treatments or other suggestions to help you.

- *Swelling in your face, arms, and legs (lymphedema):* Surgery or radiation therapy that involves your lymph nodes may cause you to retain lymph fluid and experience subsequent swelling in your face, arms, or legs. Keeping your skin clean and moisturized may help. Your physician may refer you to a physical therapist who specializes in specific types of bandages, exercises, or massage to help the fluid to drain and reduce swelling.

Coping with Your Emotions after Treatment

To help ease the transition from patient to survivor, turn to your family and friends to talk about the adjustment. Be open and express what you're feeling. Joining an organized support group also may help. Try relaxation techniques and staying active to help you cope with stress and anxiety. Tell your physician if you're feeling depressed.

During cancer treatment, relationships with friends and family often center on your illness. Learning to refocus those relationships on health and the future requires a new way of thinking. Expect a challenge as you reclaim your place in your family and circle of friends. Tell others how you feel and address their fears or questions openly. Let them know what to expect following treatment. A counselor can help if you want an impartial moderator. Many of the old stigmas associated with cancer still exist. Remind friends and coworkers that cancer isn't contagious and that research shows cancer survivors are just as productive as other workers. Adjusting to life after cancer treatment means moving past old fears and uncertainties. But it may also mean facing new ones. As you and others adapt to these changes, you may start to feel recovered.

◆ Spirituality

Spirituality is an important aspect of health care that has been frequently overlooked. Spirituality is often confused with religion. In fact, spirituality is not so much connected to a specific system of belief or worship as it is with the spirit or the soul and our search for meaning, values, and purpose in life.

Although religion may be one way of expressing spirituality, the diversity of religious beliefs and the complexities of defining spirituality add to the controversy surrounding spiritual issues in medical practice. Recent studies have shown that addressing spiritual needs can be an effective strategy for managing chronic pain or illness.

Defining Spirituality

We all have our own definition of spirituality, just as we each have our own belief systems and our individual faiths. For some, spirituality flows from religious experiences; for others, spirituality is connected to nature and feeling in tune with oneself and the universe. For still others, spirituality is expressed in music, meditation, or art. For many, spirituality encompasses all of these things.

- How do you define spirituality?
- How does spirituality affect your relationships with others? With yourself? With your God or higher power?
- What belief systems, values, and virtues do you associate with spirituality?

Spirituality and Inner Peace

Many people who are living with chronic symptoms report that they have experienced a loss of inner peace. A chronic condition may disrupt your spiritual life just as it may your physical life. Understanding and coming to terms with feelings of anger, guilt, and grief can help you to regain a sense of inner peace.

Anger

It's not surprising that many people who are living with a chronic condition are angry. It is natural to question why this has happened to you. You may be angry at your body for letting you down. If you were injured in an accident, you may be angry at whoever or whatever caused your injury. Or you may be angry at God or some higher power for allowing this to happen to you. Anger is a significant, legitimate emotion, and identifying and addressing your anger is the first step to constructive action.

If your anger is directed at circumstances within your control, dealing with those circumstances can relieve your anger and bring a sense of inner peace back into your life. However, if your anger is addressed at circumstances beyond your control, you may choose to let go of that anger as a step toward establishing or reclaiming a sense of inner peace. For those with a chronic condition, anger is often directed toward people and circumstances that are out of their control:

- Insurance company
- Employer
- Physicians/medical staff
- Family members
- Injury
- Injurer

As you analyze the source of your anger, you may find that it is misdirected. Anger at a loved one, a higher power, or yourself may in fact be misdirected anger. Understanding the source of your anger can help you to focus on constructive action.

Although anger is a valuable emotion that can lead to constructive action, studies have shown that if anger is held onto it can be physically, emotionally, and spiritually destructive. Letting anger "eat you up" not only takes away your sense of inner peace, but it may lead to depression, anxiety, self-doubt, and more anger.

Guilt

Guilt is another common emotion for people dealing with chronic conditions. You may feel as though you are somehow to blame for your condition or that if you had done something differently, you could have prevented your injury or illness. Guilt, like anger, when directed at what can't be changed, does little to increase your sense of well-being or inner peace.

By evaluating the expectations you hold for yourself, you may find that feelings of guilt stem from unrealistic expectations. Coping strategies such as positive self-talk, relaxation, role playing, and developing realistic expectations for yourself may help you to resolve feelings of guilt. As you are to others, be a friend to yourself. Direct your energy toward managing your symptoms or illness.

Grief

You may also find that you are grieving for the freedom you have lost, the things you used to be able to do, or the relationships you had before your accident or illness. Acknowledging the grief you feel can help you to move past it toward healing and coping with your symptoms.

Strategies for Spiritual Well-Being

The good news is that there are strategies that may help you establish or recover a sense of spiritual well-being just as there are strategies that may help you cope with physical symptoms. The first step toward reclaiming a sense of spiritual well-being is to recognize what actions, feelings, people, or circumstances have compromised your sense of spiritual well-being or inner peace. After you have recognized what is making you angry, anxious, nervous, or stressed, you can begin to respond effectively.

Addressing and resolving issues internally and finding peace within are ways of achieving a sense of serenity. A key to achieving internal peace often lies in finding a balance between internal reflection and communication with an objective professional, such as a member of your health care team, therapist, or clergy member.

Finally, if you decide that whatever is making you angry, anxious, nervous, or stressed is out of your control, acknowledge this and "let go." You can control your own attitudes, actions, and reactions, but you cannot control these things in others.

The following strategies may help you to regain a sense of spiritual well-being:

Understand Anger

- Give yourself permission to be angry.
- Use meditation or relaxation techniques.
- Write out your feelings and experiences in a journal.
- Find a safe place to express yourself (talk with a member of the clergy, friend, or counselor).
- Discuss feelings of anger with the appropriate party.

Improve/Maintain Relationships

- Develop listening and communication skills.
- Consider counseling as a way to improve relationships.
- Stay in touch with your health care team.
- Join a support group or faith community.

Adopt Positive Attitudes

- Focus on the positive aspects of your life.
- Use meditation and relaxation techniques, including visualization and imagery, humor, and role-playing.
- Listen to "stories of survival."
- Read inspirational stories/essays.
- Worship.
- Volunteer/participate in community service.

Ultimately, maintaining a sense of spiritual well-being is an ongoing process. Addressing issues of the soul may be difficult, but to do so may lead to inner peace.

◆ Acknowledgments

The section Cancer Survivorship: How to Cope and Thrive after Treatment is adapted from the Mayo Clinic pamphlet *Cancer Survivorship,* and the section Spirituality is adapted from the Mayo Clinic pamphlet *Spirituality.* Both pamphlets are used with the permission of the Mayo Foundation for Medical Education and Research.

10

Social Activities, Recreation, Work, and Intimacy after Cancer Treatments

◆ Will I Be Able to _____?

◆ Some Cancer Treatments Result in More Change Than Others

◆ Intimacy after Head and Neck Cancer Treatments

◆ International Association of Laryngectomees

◆ Important Points

◆ Will I Be Able to _____?

Many people who have had treatments for cancer of the larynx or tongue wonder and worry about returning to social and recreational activities they've always enjoyed. There will be many questions: Will I be able to socialize? What about using the phone? What will my boss and coworkers think? Will people in my card club accept me? Will I still be able to do woodworking? Will my grandchildren be afraid of the changes? Can I still go dancing? What about my love life? Sexuality? Kissing? Going out to eat? What about yard work? Biking? Church work? Is there any aspect of my life this disease doesn't affect? (Fig. **10–1**).

Answers to these and other questions will be different for everyone. Some answers will depend on the kind of person you've been throughout your life. Outgoing? Quiet? Social? It will depend on what "phase" in life you're in. Working? With a young family? Grandchildren? Alone? Married? It will also depend on the location and extent of your disease and the treatments you receive for it.

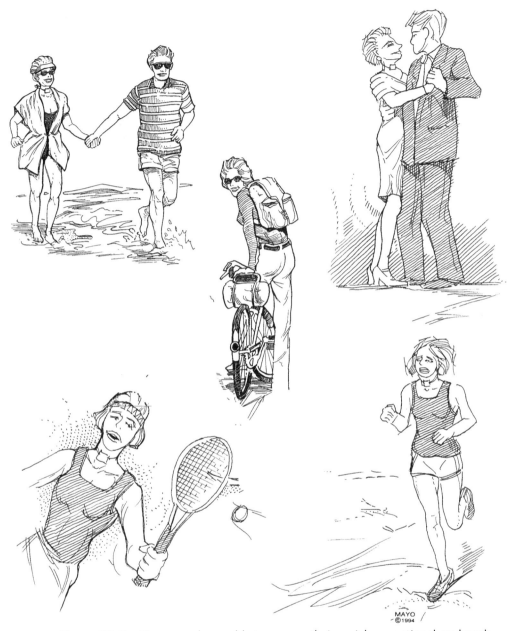

Figure 10–1   Many people are able to resume their social, recreational, and work activities after treatments for head and neck cancer. (Used with permission of the Mayo Foundation for Medical Education and Research.)

◆ Some Cancer Treatments Result in More Change Than Others

Usually surgery causes more immediate and long-lasting change in a person's swallowing, speech, and possibly breathing than radiation therapy or chemotherapy. Yet, generally speaking, most people are able to return to many of the social, recreational, and athletic activities they enjoyed before. This is true for returning to work, too, with some exceptions.

"Partial" surgeries cause problems that can usually be overcome. A person's voice can change a little or a lot by a partial laryngeal surgery. Loudness is usually reduced. A rough, hoarse, or breathy voice may linger and may or may not improve over time. Yet, people usually resume their former activities. The swallowing problems from partial surgeries typically improve, depending on the surgery. Swallowing may never get back to "normal" for every person.

In the group of people with partial surgeries are those with partial glossectomy. As described in those sections of this book, the outcome for swallowing and speech can be quite varied. Most people return to social, recreational, and work activities they participated in before treatment. But changes should be expected. For many, partial glossectomy results in distorted speech, and some foods may not be easily consumed. The person may need to speak slower to produce the best speech possible. Impaired speech may prevent a person from returning to certain types of work if there are heavy demands for public speaking or communicating over the telephone. Chewing and swallowing certain foods may be difficult or impossible after partial glossectomy. Eating a meal may take much longer and dining with others on the job during lunch breaks or business meetings may be awkward.

Perhaps those with the greatest concerns about returning to social situations, recreational activities, and work are those who have had a total laryngectomy and/or total glossectomy. These surgeries seriously compromise the ability to communicate.

For laryngectomized persons, returning to work is definitely possible, but sometimes it does not occur as quickly as some would like. Speech with an artificial larynx, esophageal voice, or tracheoesophageal puncture is usually adequate for most jobs and professions, depending on the work demands and the person's ability to master the chosen method (or methods) of alaryngeal speech.

Using an artificial larynx is usually the first, and sometimes the only, method of choice for people who have had a total laryngectomy. There are many excellent users of the artificial larynx. Yet, some laryngectomized people report that when they started using this instrument, they felt conspicuous and self-conscious, particularly when speaking in public places. After mastering the device, however, most of them give this advice to new users: "Just do it! You'll get used to it and so will everyone else!"

If the work environment is a noisy one, people using an artificial larynx or esophageal speech will face challenges. Speech with an artificial larynx is easily drowned out by noise, and esophageal speech is not as loud as the average normal voice. If the job requires the use of both hands while speaking, people who use an artificial larynx or tracheoesophageal voice without a hands-free speaking valve will face problems.

If you have had a total laryngectomy and your recreational activities or occupation requires strenuous physical activity, you may find that you need to perform these differently. Before surgery, your larynx acted as a valvelike mechanism that would "lock" air in your lungs to assist you in heavy lifting, pushing, and other activities that required your maximum or near-maximum strength. This strength may be diminished after the larynx is removed. At the same time, keep this in mind: the authors know of a woman who underwent a total laryngectomy as a young adult who later married and went on to deliver three children in the normal manner!

Reduced strength in the shoulders and arms may be the case if you have had a neck dissection. Your physician will tell you if and when you can return to work that requires upper body strength. The physician or physical therapist may suggest alternate methods that will allow you to accomplish the same activities as before.

If you breathe through a permanent tracheostoma and you return to an extremely hot and dry environment, or one that has fumes or heavy dust, some modifications will be necessary. Examples are machine or woodworking shops, construction sites, granaries, factories, and areas that are windy or have a high pollen count. Some people report the worst environments to be dry, air conditioned buildings and vehicles. Breathing difficulty can also occur during cold weather activities such as shoveling snow, and downhill and cross-country skiing. Any of these conditions can have an irritating affect on your trachea and lungs.

Discuss your work environment and recreational activities with your physician and speech pathologist. Your physician may have strong opinions about your health in these conditions. Your speech pathologist or nurse may suggest various stoma covers, devices, or treatments to help protect your trachea and lungs while you are at work.

Water sports are very dangerous after total laryngectomy. A person runs the risk of getting uncontrolled amounts of water in the lungs and of possible drowning. With some precautions, laryngectomized people can continue to enjoy fishing and boating. Watercraft must be stable and safe, and fishermen should think twice before standing up in a boat to cast out a fishing line. Ordinary life jackets and other personal flotation devices do *not* keep your tracheostoma far enough up out of the water for you to breathe safely. You will need to be aware of these dangers and take precautions because others will not understand or even think about it. If you want to swim in a pool, consider using a snorkel-like device called a Larkel. For information about this device, go to the Internet for distributors or search the Web site of the *International Association of Laryngectomees.*

In cases where very extensive cancer requires a total glossectomy, this surgery results in major changes in communication and swallowing. Speaking "on the job" or in any social or recreational event after this surgery is rarely possible. Communicating must take place in ways other than speaking, such as via e-mail, written notes, hand signals and gestures, or speech-generating devices. There are some jobs in which these nonspeaking methods of communication are adequate. For other types of work, they are not. Additionally, eating and drinking after total glossectomy with or without total laryngectomy changes dramatically.

◆ Intimacy after Head and Neck Cancer Treatments

Sexual adjustment is a common concern for people after they have had head and neck cancer treatments. They are afraid they have become sexually unattractive and unlovable. However, people are loved for their total worth. If your partner considered you lovable and sexually attractive before your operation, chances are he or she will afterward too.

There are some physical concerns of lovemaking that you may encounter as a result of cancer treatments, particularly surgery. If you have a tracheostomy, sometimes stoma odors or the sound of breathing from the stoma can be distracting. Your partner may find it disturbing to be breathed on from the stoma. There are several ways to deal with these situations. Stoma odors can be minimized by keeping the area around the stoma clean, and they may be disguised somewhat by light perfume or aftershave lotion. Using saline to clear the trachea and upper lungs of secretions may help eliminate respiratory noises. If you wear a stoma cover or a T-shirt, sounds from the stoma will be reduced slightly and your partner will not feel exhalations directly. Usually a laryngectomized person's sense of smell is not as keen as before. He or she, as well as a glossectomized person, may need to be particularly aware of their oral hygiene before intimate moments. Experimenting with different sexual positions may help relieve concerns and be enjoyable too.

Be patient with yourself and with your partner. It takes a while to adjust to these physical changes. Be as open as you can about your feelings, and try to accept your partner's honest reactions too. Many times, when one person goes through a serious illness, sharing the experience enables the couple to express their feelings about many other areas of their relationship more completely. The result is that they get to know each other better and their friendship can deepen. An honest friendship with your partner is a solid foundation for a good sex life.

◆ International Association of Laryngectomees

The International Association of Laryngectomees (IAL) is a widespread organization designed to benefit laryngectomized persons, their spouses, and family members. The IAL is composed of hundreds of local chapters, sometimes called "Lost Cord Clubs" and "New Voice Clubs."

Many of these clubs provide speech therapy, guidance and counseling, and certain equipment such as artificial larynges and stoma covers. They also offer opportunity for fellowship and support. These clubs have educational programs, group trips, holiday parties, and other social events. Each club's members decide what activities would be most beneficial for their particular membership.

Some people say the best part about joining a laryngectomee club is finding out that they're not alone. You'll be with other laryngectomized people and their spouses who have experienced the same thoughts, concerns, and feelings that you have. They'll encourage you with speech therapy. They know what it feels like to be learning to talk a different way. Many of them are probably still in the process of learning themselves. They'll have suggestions that will help you make this adjustment more easily. For many people, the greatest value of these clubs lies in the new friends they meet. For those who are not interested in support groups, getting in touch with a single member of an IAL club, such as the contact person for the club, may be all that you need or want.

For the address of the IAL club nearest you, look for the International Association of Laryngectomees on the Internet or contact your speech pathologist. If you do not have ready access to a computer, the librarian at your local public library can help you.

If there is no IAL club near you, your speech pathologist may know of other support groups in your area, or you can contact the American Cancer Society.

◆ Important Points

Whatever specific concerns you have about returning to routine life after treatment for cancer of the larynx or tongue, keep in mind these important points:

- Yes, you've changed, but you are the same person.
- Think "I'll try," not "I can't."
- Take time to recover. Cancer treatments cause most people to tire easily. Plan rest periods into your daily schedule. If you are returning to work, look into returning gradually over a period of weeks.
- Take small steps toward your goals. They add up.
- Help family, friends, and coworkers understand and become comfortable with the changes that cancer has caused in your life. Take the lead and set the pace.

Appendices

A

Communicating after Surgery and Other Treatments for Cancer of the Larynx or Tongue

The ability to communicate is essential. All treatments for cancer of the larynx or tongue can affect your speech, but surgery affects speech immediately and usually more permanently. Depending on the kind of surgery you have, before your operation you may meet with a speech pathologist, a specialist in disorders of communication, to discuss ways in which you may be able to communicate after your surgery.

Some of the methods of communication listed here may be appropriate for you soon after your surgery or later in your recovery and rehabilitation. These methods are appropriate when speaking ability is reduced after radiation therapy and chemotherapy as well:

- Attention-getting noises such as hand clapping and finger snapping (although often these are not very popular with family members and caregivers)
- Signals such as call lights or noise makers such as bells, buzzers, and horns
- Writing or printing on a paper tablet, a dry erase board, or a magic slate
- Spelling out words on an alphabet board (see Appendix J)
- Pointing to objects, pictures (see Appendix J), and printed words
- Pantomimes/hand gestures
- E-mail and Instant Messaging via computer
- Portable keyboards known as speech generating devices that "speak" what is typed
- Other voice output communication aids that speak words and phrases when pictures or symbols on a screen are touched
- A keyboard to contact and communicate with the telephone operator who will dial a number for you and relay your message to the person you are calling (refer to your telephone directory for special services for speech impaired individuals)
- Cell and mobile phones with text messaging, camera, Web access, and other capabilities
- Lifeline emergency services that respond when the person depresses a button on a communicator bracelet or pendant
- Silent-articulation speech movements that are "read" by others
- An artificial larynx (oral type or neck type) for those people without a voice, but who have sufficient tongue, lip, and jaw movement
- Tracheoesophageal puncture with voice prosthesis after total laryngectomy
- Esophageal speech after total laryngectomy

B

Speaking without a Larynx

As described in Chapter 6, speaking after total laryngectomy and extended surgeries will be very different. With the approaches available today for voice rehabilitation after laryngectomy, some form of oral communication will probably be available to you, but each of these methods will take time. Some people are disappointed that they cannot get started on a particular method of speech as soon as they would like. Some individuals may learn more than one method of speaking without a larynx, or they may start with one method and change to another. Whatever method or methods you choose, be determined to "aim high" to become excellent at that method. *It will take time, patience, practice, and perseverance* (see Appendix I).

◆ Artificial Larynx

Speech rehabilitation after total laryngectomy starts with an artificial larynx. Your speech pathologist may have demonstrated one of these devices to you before your surgery. Sometimes speech therapy with an artificial larynx can start as soon as two to three days after surgery. For others, trying an artificial larynx must be postponed due to swelling around the neck and face, pain or difficulty opening the mouth sufficiently, a swollen or stiff tongue, excessive saliva in the mouth, sore mouth, and absence of dentures.

An artificial larynx, also known as an "electrolarynx" or a "speech aid" (Figs. B–1, B–2, B–3) is a battery-powered, manufactured device used to transmit a tone or "voice" into the mouth or pharynx. These devices serve as the sound generator, and you shape the sound into words with your lips and tongue in the normal way.

There are two types of artificial larynx: oral type and neck type. Often an oral type artificial larynx is the first instrument used by a person while the neck remains swollen after surgery, particularly if a neck dissection was performed. You place a small plastic tube in your mouth that is attached to the artificial larynx. When you turn on the instrument, the tone goes through the tube directly into the mouth, and you articulate the tone into speech. When swelling in the neck reduces, you may decide to try a neck type artificial larynx. It may take some patience to find the spot on the neck where the tone is best for speech and to consistently position the instrument in that location.

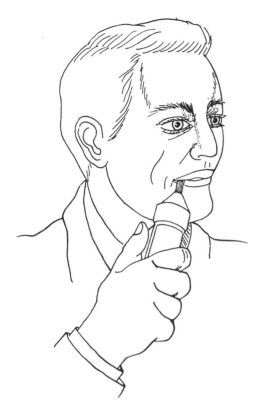

Figure B–1 An oral-type artificial larynx.

Other skills that are critical for producing understandable speech with an artificial larynx are precise articulation, a moderate speaking rate, opening your mouth to let the sound out, turning the device on and off at the right time, and use of natural phrasing. If you have dentures and/or hearing aids, wear them!

Some people comment that speech with an artificial larynx sounds "too mechanical" and "like a robot." This is true to a degree. However, laryngectomized people who become proficient at using an artificial larynx learn ways to minimize this characteristic so that it does not interfere with their ability to converse in most settings. One of the reasons for their success is that they don't settle for mediocre speech with an artificial larynx. They are determined that everything they say will be understandable to other people.

Most laryngectomized people agree that it is a good idea to own an artificial larynx and know how to use it well. Afterward, if you decide to use another method of *alaryngeal* speech, you will always have the artificial larynx as a backup method of speaking. Your speech pathologist will help guide you in selecting an artificial larynx and teach you how to use it well.

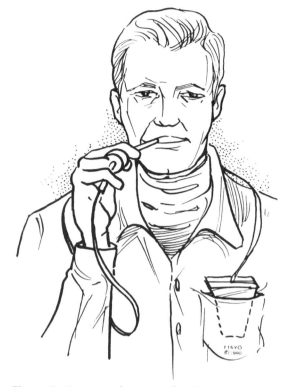

Figure B–2   An oral-type artificial larynx.

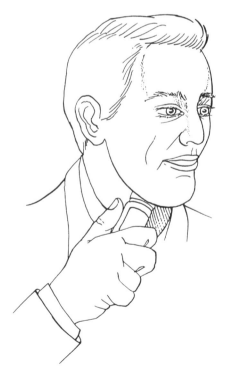

Figure B–3   A neck-type artificial larynx.

◆ Tracheoesophageal Puncture (TEP) Speech and Voice Prosthesis

Tracheoesophageal puncture (TEP) with a *voice prosthesis* is a method of speaking after total laryngectomy. This method may also be used after more extensive laryngectomy surgeries that require removal of the pharynx (throat) and esophagus (food tube) too. For these surgeries, flaps of tissue from other parts of the body — the arm, chest, or thigh — are used to reconstruct the pharynx and esophagus that have been removed. Sometimes tissue from the intestine — the jejunum — is used to replace the pharynx, or the stomach may be "pulled up" to fill in the gap where the esophagus has been removed.

To create a tracheoesophageal puncture, the surgeon makes a small opening (puncture) in the back wall of the trachea (windpipe), which is also the front wall of the esophagus (food tube). A small silicone tube known as a voice prosthesis is kept in the opening at all times to keep it from closing (Fig. B–4). The average length and diameter of a voice prosthesis are about the same as the eraser on a new pencil. One end of the prosthesis sets against the back wall of the trachea just inside the tracheostoma. This end is open to allow air to easily enter it. The other end of the prosthesis is positioned against the front wall of the esophagus and has a valve in it to keep food and liquid from entering it. If you have a TEP and a voice prosthesis is in place, when you look

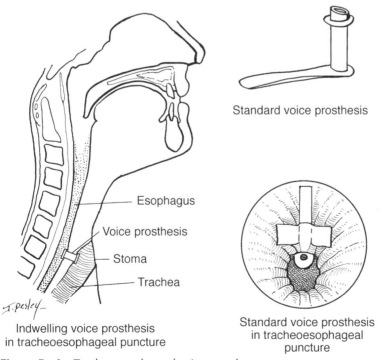

Standard voice prosthesis

Esophagus

Voice prosthesis

Stoma

Trachea

Indwelling voice prosthesis
in tracheoesophageal puncture

Standard voice prosthesis
in tracheoesophageal
puncture

Figure B–4   Tracheoesophageal voice prostheses.

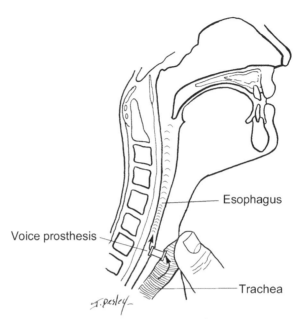

Figure B–5   Tracheoesophageal puncture with voice prosthesis (left). Producing tracheoesophageal voice for speech (right).

into your stoma in a mirror, you will see the front end of the prosthesis on the back wall of the trachea.

There are two types of voice prostheses. An indwelling prosthesis is placed and removed by your speech pathologist or physician. A standard prosthesis is one that you insert, remove, and replace yourself. Your speech pathologist will discuss with you the types of prostheses that are available and which may be best for you.

To speak with the prosthesis, you breathe in, cover the stoma with a thumb or finger, open your mouth, and then exhale (Fig. B–5). The air moves up from the lungs through the prosthesis and into the upper esophagus, which produces sound. This sound is known as TEP voice that you use for speaking. Lift your thumb or finger away from the stoma when you inhale.

Tracheoesophageal Puncture Surgery

Tracheoesophageal puncture is a relatively simple and minor surgical procedure. The surgeon can perform a TEP at the "primary" surgery when the laryngectomy is performed, or it can be performed as a "secondary" procedure some time afterward.

When would a TEP be performed for you? An assessment is made to determine if an individual is a good candidate for a TEP, and it is decided when the surgery should be performed. The timing of the TEP surgery depends on your surgeon's preferences, your speech pathologist's recommendations, your anatomy and other health and medical issues, if you have received or will receive radiation/chemotherapy treatments, your interest and motivation, and possibly other factors. If you are considering a TEP as a secondary procedure — sometime after you have healed from your laryngectomy — your speech pathologist will perform a test that can help determine what your TEP voice might sound like, and if other medical procedures may be necessary in order for you to make an easy-to-produce tracheoesophageal voice.

"Upkeep" of a Voice Prosthesis

Living with a TEP and voice prosthesis is not without its responsibilities. A prosthesis needs to be cleaned daily and sometimes more frequently. It must be removed and replaced periodically. There are decisions about what type of prosthesis is best for you. You will need a kit of cleaning supplies and other equipment close at hand so that your voice prosthesis allows air to flow through it easily at all times. Your speech pathologist will give you information on this and provide you with the training you need for developing the best voice and speaking habits possible with a prosthesis.

Like other areas of medicine, the science and art of voice restoration after laryngectomy are advancing. New procedures and products become available every year. Keep in contact with your speech pathologist and sources of current information such as the International Association of Laryngectomees to learn of these.

Tracheoesophageal Puncture + Tracheostoma Valve = "Hands-Free" Speaking

If you have a TEP with a voice prosthesis after total laryngectomy and other extended surgeries, or if you have had a near-total laryngectomy, you need to use your thumb or finger to close off the stoma when you exhale to produce voice. However, some people are able to use a device called a tracheostoma valve that allows them to speak without using a thumb or finger. The valve fits into a flexible circular housing that is attached to the skin around the stoma (Fig. B–6), or it fits into a special tube—such as the

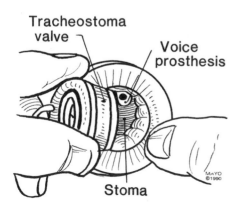

Tracheostoma valve

Voice prosthesis

Stoma

Figure B–6 Placing a tracheostoma valve over the stoma for hands-free speaking with a tracheoesophageal voice prosthesis. (Used with permission of the Mayo Foundation for Medical Education and Research.)

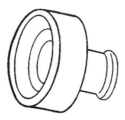

Figure B-7   The Barton-Mayo Tracheostoma Button.

Barton-Mayo Tracheostoma Button—that is inserted into the tracheostoma (Fig. B-7). The person breathes normally through the valve, and to speak he or she exhales with slightly more effort and the valve closes, acting like a finger or thumb to cover the stoma and cause air to flow through the voice prosthesis. The result is "hands-free" voice production and speech (Fig. B-8).

Not all TEP speakers or near-total laryngectomees are able to use a tracheostoma valve. With advances in surgical technique and speech

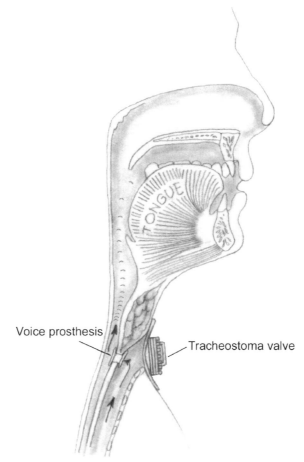

Figure B-8   A tracheostoma valve allows hands-free speaking for some people after total laryngectomy and TEP.

rehabilitation methods and products, however, these devices have become a possibility for more people. As with the voice prosthesis itself, learning to use a tracheostoma valve takes time and training, and it also requires daily maintenance. For these and other reasons, some TEP speakers choose not to use a tracheostoma valve even if they can do so.

◆ Esophageal Speech

Esophageal speech, also known as *esophageal voice,* is a method of speaking that has been used by laryngectomized people for many years. It is called esophageal voice because it is the esophagus (food tube) that produces the sound that serves as the new voice for speech. The "voice" from your esophagus sounds like a belch. However, there are important differences between speaking with esophageal voice and ordinary belching. A belch is a sound made by the esophagus when air comes up from the stomach unpredictably and in an uncontrolled way. For esophageal voice, air does not come up from the stomach. Voice is produced by sucking or pumping air from the mouth down into the upper esophagus, then immediately releasing it back up into the mouth while making speech movements with your tongue and lips (Fig. B–9). The movements necessary to produce esophageal voice are intentional, very rapid, and repeated over and over.

Becoming a good esophageal speaker takes determination and time — usually over a year of practicing many times throughout each day. It is recommended that laryngectomized persons who want to learn esophageal speech get instruction from an experienced speech pathologist or from an excellent esophageal speaker. Some laryngectomee clubs provide instruction in esophageal speech.

Some people who have had a total laryngectomy are poor esophageal speakers, or they cannot learn esophageal speech. There are several possible reasons for this. One common reason why a person cannot produce esophageal voice is because, during the surgery, the esophagus was altered in such a way that it cannot vibrate easily. Other reasons include inadequate instruction, insufficient speech practice, and social isolation that prevents frequent opportunities to speak. A speech pathologist experienced in teaching esophageal speech can discuss with you the possibilities of learning esophageal speech, as well as describe the step-by-step process that starts with making sound consistently, and then progresses to production of syllables, words, phrases, and eventually to conversational speech.

It is important to note that if a person has cancer which extends beyond the larynx to the pharynx and esophagus, and if surgery is the treatment of choice, it is highly unlikely the person will be able to learn esophageal speech that is satisfactory for everyday communication. In these cases, the tissue

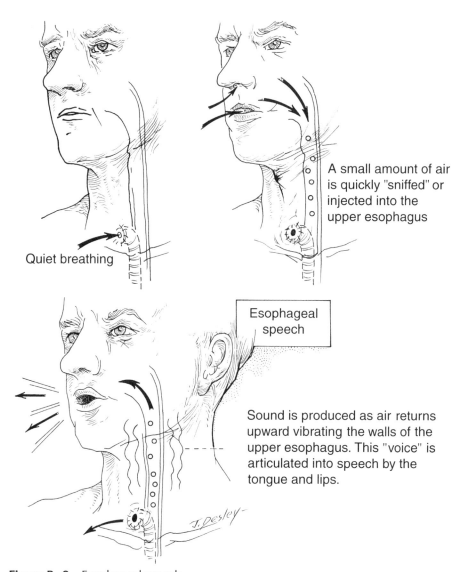

Quiet breathing

A small amount of air is quickly "sniffed" or injected into the upper esophagus

Esophageal speech

Sound is produced as air returns upward vibrating the walls of the upper esophagus. This "voice" is articulated into speech by the tongue and lips.

Figure B–9   Esophageal speech.

from another location in the body called a free flap is used to reconstruct a passage similar to the pharynx and the esophagus. The free flap tissue does not have the same "elastic" properties as the esophagus to trap air and release it in the rapid, controlled, and prolonged manner necessary for conversational speech.

C

Tube Feeding

Feeding tubes transport fluids and liquid food into your body when you can-not take them by mouth. Two types of feeding tubes, nasogastric (NG) and percutaneous gastric (PEG), are described in this appendix. Receiving food by tube is called *enteral feeding*. Only basic information about enteral feeding is provided here. Ask your physician, nurse, or dietition for specific information.

◆ Nasogastric Feeding Tube

Depending on the kind of cancer treatment(s) you receive, you may need an NG feeding tube that goes down one nostril to your upper stomach. The tube may be placed at the time of surgery or as needed at another time. Physicians vary in their preference for how long a patient uses a feeding tube, again de-pending on the needs of the patient and the cancer treatments received. Gen-erally, an NG feeding tube is in place for a few days to a few weeks. Ask your physician how this applies to you.

Tube feedings have the following advantages:

- They provide nourishment when you are unable to eat or digest food in the usual way.
- They provide balanced nutrition, including necessary vitamins, minerals, and other nutrients.
- They are fairly convenient and easy to use.

Members of your health care team — usually a nurse and dietitian — will teach you all you need to know about giving yourself liquid nutrition through your NG feeding tube. This is your opportunity to ask questions: (1) the amount of formula you need and how often you need it, (2) guidelines for storing the formula, (3) where to obtain supplies and equipment, (4) taking medication via the tube, (5) flushing the tube with water, (6) maintaining good oral care when receiving tube feedings, (7) insurance coverage issues if feedings are needed for an extended period, and (8) whom to contact after you leave the hospital if questions or problems arise concerning tube feeding. See Table C–1 for information regarding solving problems associated with na-sogastric tube feedings.

Table C – 1   Solving Problems Associated with Nasogastric Tube Feeding

Problems	Possible Causes	Solutions
Diarrhea, nausea, or cramping	Feeding solution too cold	Make sure the feeding solution is at room temperature before beginning each feeding.
	Feeding running too rapidly	Slow down the rate of feeding so that it is given over a longer period of time.
	Contaminated feeding	Check expiration date on feeding container. Check that all open bottles, cans, or mixed feedings are refrigerated and are discarded after 24 hours.
Gas or bloating	Feeding running too rapidly	Slow down the rate of feeding.
	Air in the tubing	Remove the air from the tubing by allowing the formula to run to the tip of the tubing at the beginning of each feeding. Keep feeding tube clamped between feedings.
Constipation	Too little water	Take additional water through the tube.
Thirst	Too little water	Take additional water through the tube.
Feeling of fullness	Temporary adjustment to type and volume of feeding	The sense of fullness will resolve with time. Remain sitting during and for about a half-hour after feeding. Relax and breathe slowly. The feeding may be stopped briefly until the sense of fullness is relieved.
Feeding does not run in	Clogged tubing	Relax and breathe slowly. Using a syringe, flush the tubing with a small amount of water (about one-quarter to one-half cup).
Choking feeling, coughing, gagging	Displaced nasogastric feeding tube	STOP THE FEEDING. Contact your physician.
Weight changes or swelling, sudden and/or drastic	Loss or gain of body fluids	Contact your physician.
Continuous or unusual throat discomfort	Throat irritation from nasogastric feeding tube	Contact your physician.
Skin soreness, redness at site of feeding tube insertion	Skin breakdown, irritation	Contact your physician.
Heartburn: frequent or continual	Tube irritation	Contact your physician.

◆ Care of the Nasogastric Tube

The NG tube takes the liquid nourishment down to your stomach, bypassing any areas where surgery was performed or where radiation treatments are usually directed for head and neck cancer. The tube is usually secured to your nose by tape or suture to keep it in the correct position. Keep your nostrils as clean as possible. Cleanse your nostril and lubricate the inside edge with a small amount of petroleum jelly. Cleanse crusts from the outside of the tube with small amounts of hydrogen peroxide.

If the NG tube is taped to your nose and it becomes necessary to retape it, simple bandage adhesive tapes are available, such as an NG Strip, specifically for this (Fig. C–1). A tried-and-true method of taping and securing the NG tube to the nose illustrated in Fig. C–2 works well, but is more restrictive and bulky than an NG Strip. For this method, first gently wipe any oils and tape buildup from the skin. A small amount of rubbing alcohol may help remove oils. Cut a 4-inch piece of tape as illustrated. Anchor the uncut end of the tape to your nose and wrap the split ends in opposite directions around the tube. Press the tape on firmly. If the tape tends to come off the nose before it needs to be changed, apply a liquid adhesive such as Mastisol before applying the tape.

◆ Percutaneous Endoscopic Gastrostomy Feeding Tube

For various reasons, you may need a different kind of tube than an NG tube for taking in nutrition and fluids. The most common type is a tube called a

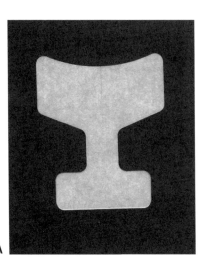
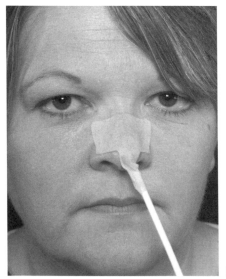

A   B

Figure C–1   A,B: A special nasogastric (NG) tape strip for securing an NG feeding tube to the nose. (Courtesy of Derma Sciences, Princeton, New Jersey.)

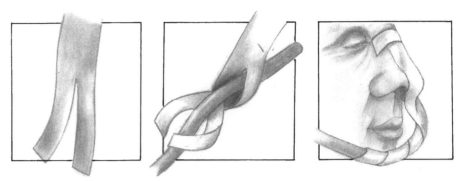

Figure C–2   A tried-and-true method of securing the NG feeding tube to the nose.

percutaneous endoscopic gastrostomy (PEG) tube (Fig. C–3). Unlike the nasogastric tube, which goes through the nose down to the stomach and is used for the short term, a PEG is a flexible tube that is inserted directly into the stomach through a small incision in the abdomen and may be used for a longer period. It provides the person with nutrition, water, and medication. A PEG does not prevent you from taking food or liquids by mouth if it is safe to do so. An extension may be placed on the tube if it must be located in the small intestine rather than the stomach.

Whether you require a temporary PEG or one for a longer term, your physician, nurse, or dietitian will explain the goals for using it and provide details of the surgical procedure for placing the tube, and will describe how to use it and how to care for the PEG site. Similar to those people who have an NG tube, if you have a PEG, thorough and frequent care of the teeth and gums is essential to keep them in good condition and to minimize odors.

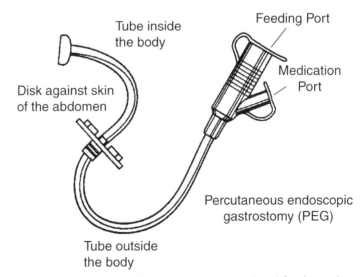

Figure C–3   A percutaneous endoscopic gastrostomy (PEG) feeding tube.

D

Swallowing Associated with Cancer of the Larynx or Tongue

◆ Your Ability to Swallow Will Be Affected by Cancer Treatments

The medical term for difficulty in swallowing is *dysphagia*. Treatments for cancer of the larynx or tongue frequently affect the ability to swallow. You may cough or choke more easily after surgery. Radiation therapy may make it difficult to swallow because of mouth and throat soreness. Advice from a speech pathologist may help you relearn to swallow after surgery. Exercises to improve movement of the tongue and throat muscles may help improve your swallowing.

◆ Tests of Swallowing Function

Your ability to swallow adequately and safely will be checked by your speech pathologist and physician. This may be done in several ways. One method is to closely observe you as you drink liquids and eat foods of different consistencies. You may be given small amounts of thin liquids, thicker liquids, and solid foods of different textures. Your ability to move each one around in your mouth, how you swallow them, how much effort it takes, and if the material was completely swallowed will be observed.

Your physician may request that the radiologist and speech pathologist perform an x-ray swallow study, often called a *videofluoroscopic swallow study* or a modified barium swallow study. If you have had surgery, the x-ray swallowing test will show if adequate healing has taken place, allowing you to take food by mouth. The swallow study will help determine if material is efficiently clearing through your throat or if some liquids and foods are going down to your lungs (*aspiration*). Sometimes after treatment for cancer, the sensation in the throat is impaired and a person does not cough when liquids and food go down the wrong tube. This will appear on the x-ray study. This evaluation helps determine which consistencies are swallowed most efficiently and if there are certain techniques you can use to improve your swallowing.

Another test that provides a different view and different information about the swallowing mechanism is called the fiberoptic endoscopic evaluation of swallowing and sensory test (FEESST). During this test, either your speech pathologist or your physician will pass a thin, lighted flexible scope through the nose and down into the throat. A recording is usually made as you swallow liquids and foods. This test shows how well foods and liquids pass through your throat and if they are leaking down the trachea toward your lungs.

◆ Modifying the Consistency of Foods and Liquids Taken by Mouth

> Important note: If you have not been taking food by mouth it is important that your physician gives approval before you can begin eating by mouth and before a feeding tube is removed.

Many people with cancer of the larynx or tongue must change their diet before surgery, radiation therapy, or chemotherapy to reduce coughing, discomfort, the risk of aspiration, and weight loss. After these treatments, the *consistency* or texture of foods and liquids you take by mouth must change, at least in the beginning. This section provides suggestions for modifying the consistency of your foods and liquids.

Guidelines for obtaining the desired consistency for a liquid diet, semi-solid diet, and soft diet are listed below. Your speech pathologist, physician, and dietitian may be quite definite about which diet consistencies are right for you at any particular time. Do not make changes in the consistency of your liquids or foods unless your medical team gives you the "green light" to do so.

◆ Liquid Consistency Diets

A liquid diet contains liquids and other foods that are processed in a blender until they are of smooth consistency. There are no distinct pieces of food, and no chewing is required. Usually liquid is added to the blenderized food until it is the desired consistency. Liquids that are too runny can be thickened with a powdered food starch thickener. Here are four consistency levels for liquids:

- *Thin liquids:* These include water, coffee, tea, soda, ices, milk, juice, or anything that will liquify in the mouth within a few seconds.
- *Nectar-like:* Apricot or peach nectar, or thin liquids thickened to nectar consistency. Consult your dietitian about the consistency of commercial liquid nutrition products such as Ensure.
- *Honey-like:* Liquids that are thickened to honey consistency.
- *Spoon-thick:* Liquids that are thickened to a pudding consistency. Examples are pureed meat, mashed and thinned potato. Commercial thickener can be added to beverages to obtain this level of thickness.

◆ Semisolid, Soft, and Solid Consistency Diets

Like liquids, diet recommendations for food are based on consistency. Your dietitian may provide you with more explanation, menus, and printed material concerning these food consistencies. Here are four consistency levels for food:

- *Pureed:* These foods are blenderized, cohesive, and pudding-like. A meal could consist of pureed chicken, mashed potatoes with gravy, pureed cooked carrots, applesauce, and chocolate pudding.
- *Mechanically altered:* These foods are cohesive, moist, and soft textured. These require some chewing ability and include ground or finely diced meats, "fork mashable" soft-cooked vegetables, soft ripe or canned fruit, and some moistened cereals. Most bread products, crackers, and other dry foods are excluded. A meal could consist of scrambled egg, pancake with syrup, cold cereal with milk, banana, and orange juice.
- *Advanced/soft-solid:* These foods require more chewing ability and include easy-to-cut meats, vegetables, and fruits. Hard, crunchy vegetables and fruits, and sticky foods are excluded from this group. A meal could consist of vegetable soup, shredded lettuce salad with dressing, turkey sandwich with mayonnaise, fresh ripe melon, and chocolate cookie with no nuts.
- *Regular:* This group contains any solid textures.

◆ Definitions of Food Preparation Terms

Often people have different ideas of what certain food preparation terms mean. When discussing food preparation with your dietitian, make certain you understand the terms and that you are using them to mean the same thing the dietitian means. Here are definitions of commonly used terms:

- *Puree:* A smooth paste or thick liquid. There are no distinct pieces of food. A puree is made by processing foods in a blender with added liquid. Chewing is not necessary.
- *Blenderize:* To process food in a blender. The particle size will vary according to the length of time left in the blender. The thickness will vary according to the amount of liquid added.
- *Ground:* Ground foods have been put through a food grinder to break down fiber and connective tissue. There are small (approximately one-eighth inch) but distinct pieces. Little chewing is required.
- *Chop:* Chopped foods have been cut in pieces smaller than one-quarter inch. Some chewing is necessary.
- *Dice:* Diced foods have been cut in pieces of approximately one-quarter inch. Chewing is necessary.

◆ Therapy for Swallowing Problems Associated with Cancer of the Larynx and Tongue

Difficulty swallowing (dysphagia) is a common problem associated with cancer of the larynx or tongue before, during, and after medical treatments. Swallowing difficulty may be one of the first signals that cancer is present in the mouth or throat. During radiation therapy or chemotherapy treatments, swallowing may become more difficult. After these treatments, as well as after surgery, swallowing ability may improve. For some people, swallowing problems may actually increase over time even after successful cancer treatments. The swallowing outcome depends on where the cancer is located, the size of the cancer, and the course of treatment that is taken. Due to these complicated variables, you will benefit from consultation with a speech pathologist who specializes in swallowing disorders and swallowing therapy to help you with the actual swallowing of food and liquids soon after cancer of the larynx or tongue is diagnosed.

A swallowing therapy program is carefully developed with consideration of six important components:

1. The structures and movements involved in normal swallowing (see Chapter 2)
2. Careful study and diagnosis of the problem (See Tests of Swallowing Function, above)
3. Determining if the diet must be altered in consistency to reduce or prevent problems (see Modifying the Consistency of Foods and Liquids Taken by Mouth, above)
4. Determining if certain techniques or maneuvers improve ability to swallow (see below)
5. Determining if exercises can reduce or prevent swallowing problems (see Appendix E)
6. The timing of swallowing therapy in relationship to head and neck cancer treatments, and any other factors

Swallowing therapy is based on each person's unique circumstances. The swallowing techniques and maneuvers listed below are known to help people with dysphagia due to cancer of the larynx or tongue before, during, or after various medical treatments. Often these therapy techniques must be modified to meet each person's individual needs. Your speech pathologist will be your guide as you practice various swallowing techniques—some by themselves, some in combination with others, and some in combination with certain food consistencies—to determine which are most beneficial for you. If you are having problems aspirating foods or liquids, some of these techniques are *not* for you! *Again, follow your speech pathologist's and physician's recommendations carefully for a swallowing therapy program that is best for you.*

- Moving the tongue differently or more vigorously to push food and liquid toward the back of the mouth and throat
- Holding the head in a certain position, such as with the chin tipped toward the chest or with the head turned to the left or right, to help close off the airway and direct foods and liquids on the correct pathway as they are swallowed
- Swallowing with more effort
- Swallowing more than once
- Holding the breath while swallowing
- Bearing down while swallowing
- Intentionally coughing after swallowing
- Alternating swallows of food and liquid
- Taking smaller sips or bites
- Using specially designed equipment such as a cup that releases a limited amount of liquid when it is tipped, or a spoon-like utensil or chopsticks that help place food back further in the mouth when tongue function is reduced or absent

◆ Summary

A speech pathologist may be able to help with the swallowing difficulties you encounter as a result of cancer of the larynx or tongue. Since every person is different, every "prescription" for swallowing therapy will be different. One prescription does not fit all.

E

Speech and Swallowing Exercises

Exercising the lips, tongue, and jaw may help improve speech and swallowing problems due to surgery, radiation therapy, chemotherapy, or any combination of these treatments for cancer of the larynx or tongue. Also, if you have had a form of partial laryngectomy, exercises for the remaining larynx may improve voice production and swallowing.

Speech and swallowing exercises often focus on range of motion; that is, moving the lips, tongue, and jaw to extreme positions and holding those positions for a short period to gently stretch and sometimes strengthen muscles, before relaxing. Practicing oral postures and movements for particular speech sounds, for example the /t/ and /k/ sounds, and exaggerating and "freezing" various steps of the swallowing process have also been found to improve speech and swallowing outcomes. Besides focusing your attention on the positions, movements, and processes in speech and swallowing, frequent exercising may increase the accuracy and speed of the movements.

Usually speech and swallowing exercises can begin as soon as there has been adequate healing after surgery. For those undergoing either or both radiation therapy and chemotherapy, exercises can begin any time during the course of treatments, but often these are started just before or early in the treatments. Again, every person is different, and your speech pathologist will probably be communicating with your physicians about these decisions.

Your speech pathologist will prescribe the exercises for you and demonstrate how to do them. Working in front of a mirror, at least in the beginning, may help you know if you are practicing the movements correctly. How long or how many times a person performs a set of exercises will vary. Research has shown positive results when oral exercises are done 10 times a day for five to 10 minutes each time. As a general rule, start doing exercises slowly and gently for brief periods and gradually increase the number of repetitions and amount of practice time. Try to use smooth, nonjerky movements. Using the mirror will help you see what part you are moving and how much. Use a flashlight to see movement inside the mouth.

As with any exercise program, it is up to you to follow through with the exercise routine that is recommended. You need to put some effort into these exercises and "push" a little. You may experience fatigue or slight aching in muscles for a while. This is to be expected. However, the old adage "no pain, no gain" does not apply here. If a particular movement causes you pain, don't push quite so hard, or discontinue the exercise until you discuss it with your speech pathologist or physician.

Important note: Be certain to discuss your individual situation with your speech pathologist and physician before embarking on an exercise program.

Range of motion exercises are for specific muscle groups and their functions. They are of help for some people but not for everyone undergoing treatment for cancer of the head and neck. The movements shown here are examples. There is nothing special or magic about them. Your speech pathologist will help you analyze your situation to develop a set of range of motion exercises that fit your particular circumstances.

Start by asking yourself, "What parts of my mouth or throat do I need to move better to maintain or improve my voice, speech, or my ability to chew, move food around in my mouth, and swallow?" Exercises for the lips, tongue, jaw, and remaining larynx are described on the following pages. Illustrations accompany some of the printed descriptions. The order or sequence in which you perform these movements is not important, although it may be easier to keep track of what you are moving and how many times you do it if you stick with a certain routine.

It should be fine for you to develop your own variations of these movements. Keep in mind that you are focusing on the best range of motion of all the parts of your mouth and throat for the best speech, chewing, and swallowing you can do.

Even if you are unable to make the movements described and pictured here, keep working at it. Think about how the movement is supposed to look, think positively, and in your mind envision yourself accomplishing the movement.

One final recommendation: If you cannot produce specific speech sounds, for example, the /k/ or /s/ sounds, ask your speech pathologist for suggestions on how to pronounce them or how to make sounds that are similar to them.

◆ Exercises for the Lips

Obtaining adequate closure of the lips is essential for making certain speech sounds such as /p/, /b/, and /m/. The lips also play an important role in the swallowing process. They prevent saliva, food, and liquids from running out of the mouth, and they help move this material to the back of the mouth to be swallowed. Even if you cannot achieve the positions and movements shown in the drawings, envision yourself accomplishing them as you practice.

- Press your lips together and keep them sealed as tightly as possible. Hold this position for a few seconds (Fig. E–1).
- With teeth closed, spread your lips as widely as possible, as if to show all your teeth in a "big fake smile." Feel your lips stretch. For a variation of this exercise, open your jaw slightly (Fig. E–2).
- Put your lips together and push them forward into a tight pucker. Hold this posture for a few seconds, then "point" your puckered lips to the right and hold, then to the left and hold (Fig. E–3).

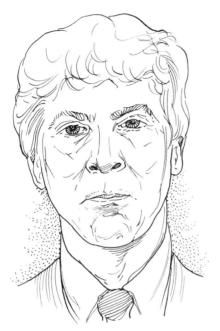

Figure E–1

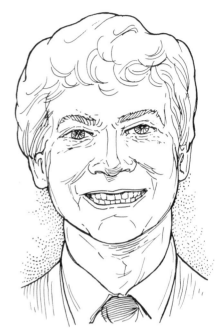

Figure E–2

- Hold your lips together and shape them into a tight circle as if you are saying the word *oh* (Fig. E–4). Hold this position for a few seconds, then "point" your rounded lips to the right and hold, then to the left and hold.

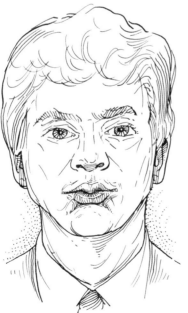

Figure E–3

◆ Exercises for the Tongue

The tongue plays a critical role in producing speech and for preparing and moving food and liquids in the mouth for swallowing. Surgery on the tongue affects its size, strength, mobility, and speed. Radiation therapy to the tongue and surrounding areas and chemotherapy treatments have similar effects on it. Use a mirror when performing tongue exercises to help you see if it is your tongue that is moving and not your jaw. If your tongue doesn't look like, or cannot be positioned like, what is shown in the drawings, ignore the drawings and practice anyway!

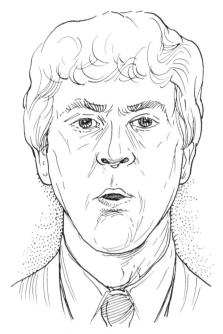

Figure E–4

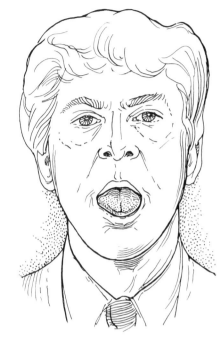

Figure E–5

- Stick your tongue straight out of your mouth as far as possible and hold it (Fig. E–5). Pull it back in. Keep moving it as far back as it will go. Hold it there for a few seconds, then stick it out of your mouth again.

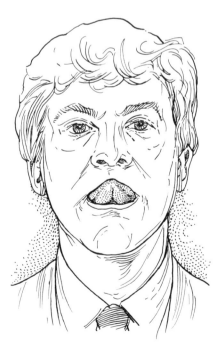

Figure E–6

- Stick your tongue straight out, then raise the tip up toward your nose (Fig. E–6). In the beginning, you might use a tongue depressor to help direct your tongue. Then, stick your tongue straight out and point it down toward your chin.

- Poke your tongue into your right cheek as far as possible (Fig. E–7). Hold it and, if you can, wiggle it around in your cheek. Then move your tongue to the left side and poke it into the cheek. Wiggle it. For a variation of this exercise, poke your tongue into your right cheek and resist it by pushing the bulge in your cheek with your finger. Do the same on the left side.

- With your mouth closed or slightly open, raise up your tongue tip (or as much of the tongue as possible) to the roof of the mouth (Fig. E–8) and slowly glide it back along the roof of your mouth as far back as you can. Then reverse this movement.

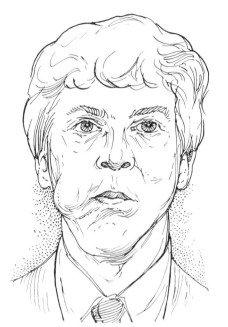

Figure E–7

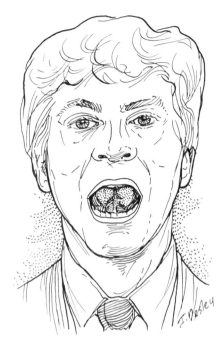

Figure E–8

- There are many variations to these tongue exercises. Figs. E–9 and E–10 show examples of using a tongue depressor to "push" against with the tongue. These and similar resistance exercises may help increase strength and improve positioning and movement of the tongue.

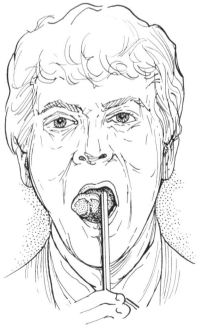

Figure E–9

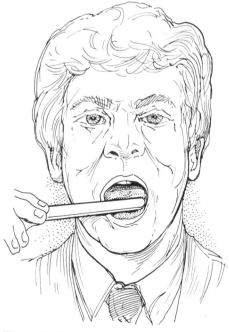

Figure E–10

◆ Exercises for the Jaw

Jaw movement is important for chewing food, making speech sounds, and letting voice and speech "out." Sometimes surgery, radiation therapy, and chemotherapy can affect the jaw so that it can hardly open. These exercises and variations of them are to help keep the jaw mobilized and increase its range of motion. Do not exercise to the point of pain.

- Open your mouth as far as possible (Fig. E–11). If this causes pain, don't open it as far—open it to and hold it at the point just before discomfort. Hold the open position for several seconds, then close your jaw and relax.
- Use a wooden tongue depressor on its side to help keep your jaw open (Fig. E–12). If your jaw does not open very far, start with one tongue depressor or two tongue depressors taped together and place them lying flat between your front teeth or back teeth to help keep your jaw open. Add more tongue depressors as your jaw is able to open more. Ask your speech pathologist about other devices that exercise the jaw and measure the amount of jaw openness.
- A red rubber catheter can be used to practice chewing. This type of catheter is sturdy and soft and will not injure your teeth or mouth. Hold one end in your hand and gently chew on the other end. Avoid attempting to bite off a piece of the catheter. Ask your speech pathologist or nurse for several red rubber catheters.
- Jut your jaw out forward as far as possible and hold that position. Relax before repeating.
- Jut your jaw out forward, then slide it as far to the right as possible and then as far to the left as possible. Go slowly.
- Jut your jaw out forward, and rotate it clockwise, then counterclockwise.

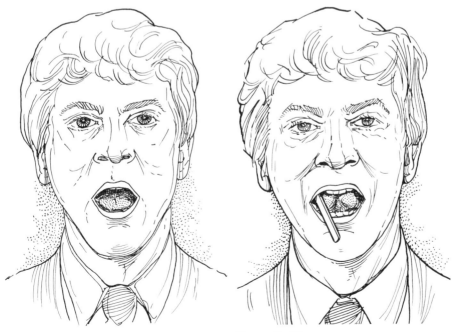

Figure E–11   **Figure E–12**

◆ Exercises for the Larynx and Partial Larynx

The larynx or "voice box" produces voice for speech and it protects the airway from food and liquid entering the lungs during swallowing. If you have had radiation therapy or chemotherapy for laryngeal cancer or a form of partial laryngectomy—part of the larynx is removed, but part of the larynx is preserved—your voice may be breathy and rough sounding and monotone, and it may tire easily. After surgery, swallowing may be a problem, particularly with thin liquids, because there isn't enough tissue to completely close off the airway. Coughing, aspiration, respiratory illness, and anxiety may result.

The purpose of exercises for the larynx after partial laryngectomy surgeries, radiation therapy, or chemotherapy is to achieve better voice quality and to improve swallowing ability. *It is particularly important before starting any exercises for the larynx that you consult your physician and speech pathologist* to determine which exercises are most therapeutic for you, how best to perform them, and when in the course of your medical treatments they should be practiced.

- Say the vowel /ah/ with effort so it is "loud and long." Pushing or pulling against something stable while doing this may be helpful.
- Coughing, holding your breath, clearing your throat, and/or grunting may help improve closure of the remaining larynx.
- Sliding up and down the musical scale to reach your highest and lowest notes may promote more pitch variation in the voice, and there may be certain tones in your vocal range that have a better sound quality than others. In addition, this exercise may increase muscle movement to raise up the partial larynx for improved closure during swallowing. As you gently and slowly practice this exercise, without excessive effort and strain, think about the up and down movement of the larynx in your throat and how many different notes you can produce. Do not think of this as singing or be disappointed in your voice. If you enjoy singing, however, do it. Singing, too, can be good exercise for the larynx after partial laryngectomy.

F

Living with a Permanent Tracheostomy

Important note: If you have had a near-total laryngectomy, total laryngectomy, or total laryngectomy and additional surgery such as on the tongue, pharynx, or esophagus, your tracheostomy will be permanent. This appendix is intended for you. *There are other laryngeal problems and breathing conditions that require the use of a long-term or permanent trach tube. The information in this section is not intended for those conditions. Consult your physician for information on managing the trach tube for your situation.*

◆ The Ins and Outs of a Trach Tube

Most people who are about to undergo a near-total laryngectomy or total laryngectomy are shocked when they learn they will be permanently breathing through an opening in their neck. They're shocked again when they hear they will need to wear a tube in the opening, at least for a period of time, in order for it to heal and stay open and large enough for easy breathing. And, when they hear they must learn to remove the tube, clean it, and then place it back into the stoma on a daily basis, the most common response is, "I'll never be able to do that!" However, this usually isn't the case. After a few training sessions with an ear, nose, and throat (ENT) nurse or other caregiver, the anxieties and fears diminish, and these persons learn to do all the necessary stoma care and hygiene within a few days of the surgery.

◆ How to Clean a Metal Tracheostomy Tube

It is important to keep the trach tube clean. The inner *cannula* of the trach tube should be cleaned as needed. The outer cannula will probably only need to be cleaned once a day. Consider using the following method of cleaning your trach tube if your surgeon or ENT nurse has not recommended another way. To do this, you will need the following:

- An inside tube brush
- A hand brush
- Mild liquid dish detergent
- Hydrogen peroxide (3% solution)
- Warm tap water

The cleaning brushes will probably be given to you by your nurse. If not, you can buy them from a medical supply store or drug store. Use any mild liquid dish detergent. Hydrogen peroxide can be purchased at a drug store and most supermarkets. Sterile equipment isn't necessary for cleaning the trach tube unless you are instructed otherwise. If you follow these steps, you'll be able to keep the tube sufficiently clean.

1. Wash your hands thoroughly with soap and water, then dry them.
2. Remove the entire tube (both inner and outer cannulas) from the stoma and throw away the soiled sponge dressing. A spongelike dressing is preferred over a plain gauze pad, which can become stringy and does not absorb as well. Discard the neck strap with Velcro fastener tabs or twill tie tapes if they are soiled.
3. Use the hand brush, warm water, and detergent to clean the outside of the inner and outer cannulas. Rinse thoroughly. If crusty secretions remain on

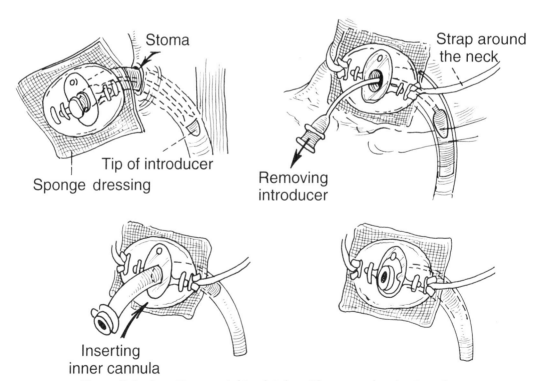

Figure F–1   Inserting a metal trach tube with sponge dressing into the stoma.

the tube, pour hydrogen peroxide directly over the tube before cleaning it again with soap and water.

4. Rinse the tubes well. If crusty secretions remain, put hydrogen peroxide on the tube brush and scrub the inside of the tubes again. Rinse the tubes completely with water to remove the hydrogen peroxide.

5. Clean the brushes to remove all the mucus and shake the tubes dry.

To put the outer cannula of the trach tube back into the stoma easily, wet it with water or lubricate it with a small amount of water-based lubricant such as Surgilube or KY Jelly. Use the inserter/introducer as necessary for comfortable insertion into the stoma (Fig. F–1).

◆ Using a Sponge Dressing with the Trach Tube

Immediately after near-total or total laryngectomy and probably for a month or so afterward, you may be wearing a sponge dressing under your tracheostomy tube to absorb secretions. Your nurse will show you how to do this and supply you with some sponges and neck straps before you leave the hospital. If not, these materials are available in most pharmacies. Ask for 4- × 4-inch sponge pads. These pads come precut to fit around the back of your trach tube, or perhaps your nurse will show you how to cut sponges yourself. Uncut sponges are less expensive than precut ones. The easiest way to use this dressing is to remove the trach tube completely, put the dressing around the tube, and then replace the tube in tracheostoma.

◆ Using a Foam Neck Strap or Twill Tie Tapes with the Trach Tube

As long as you have a tracheostomy tube, you will need to hold it in place with a foam neck strap or twill tie tapes. You will be shown how to use these when you are in the hospital.

Some people prefer a neck strap made of foam material with Velcro tabs that fasten onto the trach tube. These are comfortable and easy to use, and they do not entail raising one's arms behind one's head for tying (which may be difficult for those who have had a neck dissection). Others may choose twill ties because they are not as warm around the neck as foam straps. Also, some foam neck straps are too short for large necks, whereas twill ties can be cut to any length necessary. Some reuse of the foam neck strap or twill tie tapes may be possible if they are thoroughly rinsed and dried; however, they should be replaced frequently.

◆ Tracheostoma Hygiene

Keep your tracheostoma clean. Gently cleanse the skin around the tube with mild soap and water. If kept free of secretions, the skin will not become as irritated. Ask your physician if a lubricant around your stoma will help protect it and prevent crusting. Sometimes an antibiotic ointment is used around the stoma to help promote healing. Change the sponge dressing under the tube when it becomes soiled. This may help prevent the skin from becoming irritated and will reduce or prevent stoma odors.

◆ Use of Saline

Physicians and nurses often encourage patients to use saline in their tracheostoma to increase humidity and help reduce dried mucus in the trachea and lungs. Saline thins thick secretions and loosens dried pieces and helps you cough out this material. Many people report that saline helps them breathe easier and feel better immediately. Some do not like to use saline because it makes them cough, which it does. However, many people say when they use saline and cough out thick mucus that was trapped in the trachea and lungs, they cough less afterward.

Saline comes in large containers as well as in convenient, small plastic single-use vials that can be purchased at a pharmacy. A prescription is necessary in some areas. Or you can make your own saline solution and squirt it into your stoma with an eyedropper.

Saline can be made by mixing one-eighth teaspoon of salt in one cup of boiled tap water or distilled water. Add the salt to the water while it is hot to help it dissolve. Cool the solution and pour some into a small clean bottle with an eyedropper top that is easy to carry around. Store the remaining saline solution in a clean jar in the refrigerator. Discard unused saline after one week and make new solution.

Use the contents of a vial or an eyedropper of saline down your trachea in the morning and at night and throughout the day as needed to aid in humidity and easier breathing. Use two vials or several full eyedroppers at a time if needed. If you carry saline in a pocket close to your body, it will warm to your body temperature and may be more comfortable to use than cold solution.

◆ Coughing Out Secretions

Laryngectomized people remove secretions from the trachea and lungs by breathing deeply, then forcefully coughing them out the stoma. Using saline will help soften and liquify the secretions so they can be coughed out more easily.

Remember to hold a tissue at your tracheostoma when you cough. If secretions don't move "up and out" very readily, you may find the following method helpful. While in a seated position with knees apart, take in a deep breath, then lean forward and cough a few times vigorously. It may help to push on your abdomen at the moment you cough. Have plenty of tissues at hand. Repeat and relax when necessary. Coughing from this position can be a very productive method of removing secretions. However, because some sphincter action is no longer present after total laryngectomy, this position may cause the contents of your stomach to "roll out" of your stomach and esophagus and into your mouth and nose, particularly if you have eaten or drunk recently! This is not uncommon. If it occurs, be calm, and try again when your stomach is not as full.

◆ Moist Air for Breathing after Tracheostomy

After near-total or total laryngectomy, your nose and mouth no longer function to warm, humidify, and filter the air you breathe. As described earlier, dry air can cause plugs of mucus to form in the trachea and lungs. It can also cause the windpipe to become excessively dry, crusty, and irritated. These problems can cause coughing and make breathing difficult. Increasing the humidity of the air you breathe may help.

You can increase the moisture in the air of your home by running a warm humidifier or vaporizer in the main living areas during the day and in your bedroom at night. Some people say that when dry conditions seem especially severe, they stand over the humidifier and inhale the air more directly or they spend more time in the shower to loosen dried mucus and cough it out. Use fresh water or cooled boiled water in your humidifier and follow the manufacturer's recommendations for cleaning the humidifier at regular intervals.

Some "neck breathers" don't leave the house without a small pump bottle to spray a mist of plain tap water or distilled water directly into their tracheostoma to increase humidity and decrease dryness. Others prefer to dampen their *stoma cover* with water for increased moisture.

◆ Wearing a Stoma Cover

When you are not actively cleaning your stoma or bathing, your stoma should be shielded by a "stoma cover" (Fig. F–2). A stoma cover looks like a bib or dickey. It ties behind the neck or has straps with Velcro for easy fastening and removal. It serves as a filter to prevent dust from getting into the lungs. It keeps out other foreign materials like hair, liquids, or food. Also, depending on the material it is made of, a stoma cover can help increase the temperature and moisture of the air you breathe in.

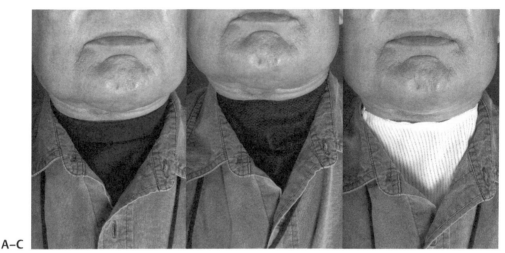

A–C

Figure F–2   A–C: Examples of stoma covers.

There are many types of stoma covers available commercially. Cloth or knit stoma covers worn under a shirt can look like a casual crew neck T-shirt or a dressier mock turtleneck. Some are made of a layer or two of thin fabric. Others are made of foam or a combination of cloth and foam. A stoma cover can be a 2- × 2-inch patch of foam sheeting that tapes to the skin directly above the stoma, although this type is too small if you are wearing a trach tube.

Wearing a stoma cover at all times is important whether your activity is indoors or outdoors. The type of stoma cover you use may change over time or with your activity. A cover of tightly woven fabric or two layers of protection may be of choice when pollen count is high or if an activity takes place in a dusty environment. A cover of light, loosely woven fabric or thin foam may suffice under other conditions. Multiple layers may be necessary to cover the stoma in freezing temperatures.

There are important reasons for wearing a stoma cover other than for filtering, warming, and humidifying the air you breathe. When you wear a stoma cover your stoma is not visible and does not attract the unwanted attention of others. Equally important, a stoma cover prevents secretions from flying across the room or at someone when you cough unexpectedly!

Stoma covers of one type may meet the needs of one laryngectomized person but may be inconvenient or uncomfortable for another. Experiment with different kinds of stoma covers to discover what works best for you.

Generally speaking, the longer a person has been laryngectomized, the less mucus he or she produces, and coughing decreases. As a result, some laryngectomees need not be concerned about mucus ruining their clothing. They can wear ordinary pullover or button-up shirts to cover the stoma, or they can wear scarves, pendants, bolo ties, and other creative neckwear over the stoma. One woman who has been active in the International Association of

Laryngectomees for many years is well known for wearing a beautiful seashell on a chain that covers her stoma!

◆ Heat and Moisture Exchangers

Using a cover of some sort over the stoma, such as a biblike cloth cover, a foam patch, a dickey, a scarf, or even a T-shirt that covers the stoma, helps to simulate some of the functions of the nose and mouth, at least to a degree. However, greater noselike results can be achieved when a *heat and moisture exchanger* (HME) is used (Fig. F–3). An HME fits closely over the stoma and you breathe in and out through it. It contains foam or other materials that serve as filters. Research has shown that HMEs not only filter air but also capture the heat and moisture of the air when the person exhales, and then immediately return that heat and moisture to the lungs when the person inhales. An HME helps keep the air in the lungs at a higher temperature that is closer to the temperature as when the person was breathing through the nose and mouth before surgery.

Favorable results have been reported by laryngectomized people who wear HMEs. Some say they produce less mucus in their lungs, and they cough less when they use an HME. Others say they have more energy, they sleep better at night, and their airway doesn't dry out as much. The respiratory system also benefits from an HME over the tracheostoma because it provides some resistance during breathing that is similar to breathing naturally through the nose and mouth.

The benefits of wearing an HME often do not occur immediately, and results vary from person to person. Some laryngectomized people try an HME, but for various reasons, choose not to continue wearing one.

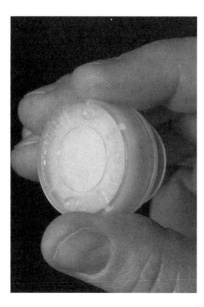

Figure F–3   An example of a heat and moisture exchanger (HME). (Courtesy of InHealth Technologies, Carpinteria, California. *www.inhealth.com.*)

◆ Showering

Showering is not usually a problem for people who are breathing through a tracheostomy tube or stoma, but a few adjustments are necessary. First, it is important for all "neck breathers" to be cautious around water, particularly if it is of any depth, such as in a bathtub, hot tub, swimming pool, or lake. Given the opportunity, water will pour directly through the tracheostoma and into the lungs. Drowning would be a real possibility.

However, there is little concern about showering if you take precautions. Remember that small amounts of water and the warm mist of the shower entering the stoma will help you clear out thick secretions.

Here are some suggestions. Adjust the showerhead so that the stream of water hits your body below the level of your stoma. When you need to rinse your head or neck area, try cupping your hand over the stoma, or wring out your washcloth and place it over the stoma. Try rinsing your hair with your back to the showerhead so the majority of the water goes down your back. Some people like to use a hand-held shower for more control of the spray. Others prefer to use a child's plastic bib over the stoma or one of the shower guards that are available from some laryngectomy equipment outlets or medical supply houses (Fig. F–4).

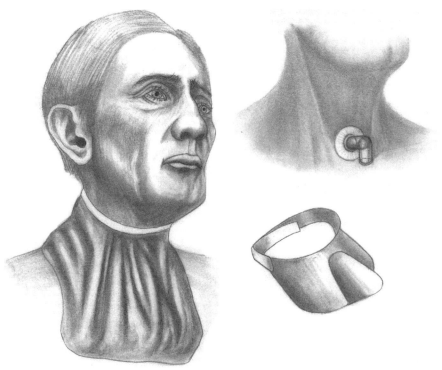

Figure F–4   Samples of shower guards.

◆ Leaving the Tracheostomy Tube Out

All tracheostomas are not alike. One person's stoma may stay the same size as the day the surgeon created it. Another person's tracheostoma may shrink in a few hours' time from the size of a nickel or a penny to the diameter of a pencil eraser. Some stomas even "close down" in just a few hours, making breathing very difficult and even requiring emergency intervention. These individual variations may be due to the surgeon's technique of creating the stoma, or changes in tissues of the neck as a result of radiation therapy, or for unknown reasons.

Many laryngectomized people no longer need to wear a trach tube after a few days to a few months after their surgery. Some people require longer use of a trach tube if they undergo radiation therapy or chemotherapy after surgery. A small percentage of people need to wear a trach tube most of the time or all of the time on a permanent basis.

Your physician will discuss with you the schedule for wearing the trach tube and when you may begin the gradual process of leaving it out. *It is in your best interest that you do not make the decision to leave the trach tube out on your own. Get your physician's approval first!*

If your physician says it is time to try leaving the trach tube out, he or she may instruct you in a procedure similar to this one: Take the trach tube out and leave it out for an hour. Then notice whether you feel resistance when you put the tube back in the stoma. Resistance indicates that the stoma has shrunk during the period the tube was out. This means that your body is not yet ready for you to leave the tube out permanently. Eventually, you'll probably be able to leave it out for longer periods of time, and then leave the tube out all day and still be able to replace it easily at night. When this happens several evenings in a row, you may leave the tube out all night. Do not leave it out at night until you have reached this point and your physician gives approval.

◆ Using a Stoma Vent

If your stoma tends to shrink slightly or it seems to close off somewhat when you turn your head to the side or tip your chin toward your chest, but you don't need a trach tube in all the time, a silicone tube called a "stoma vent," "laryngectomy tube," "stoma button," or "stoma stud" may provide the support necessary to keep it at the desired size and prevent contracture. Your physician or ENT nurse will tell you if and when you are a candidate for one of these.

Several types of stoma vents and similar tubes are available. Most are light, pliable tubes that come in various lengths and diameters. Figure F–5 shows how to insert one type of stoma vent. Most people appreciate the switch from a metal or plastic trach tube to a stoma vent. Usually they are comfortable and easy to clean, and some don't require a strap around the neck to keep them in place.

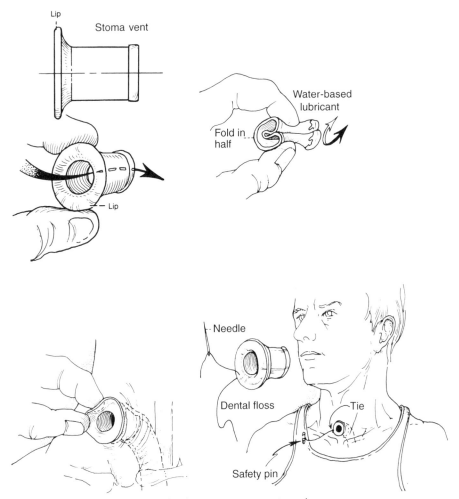

Figure F–5   Inserting a flexible plastic stoma vent into the stoma.

◆ Fear of Suffocating

Some people are afraid they might suffocate in their sleep if they place blankets or sheets over their trach tube or stoma. Practically speaking, you don't need to worry about suffocating. Your tracheostomy opening is large enough to obtain all the air you need to breathe easily, and you can usually breathe through the covers. But, if they should obstruct your breathing while you are sleeping, you will do exactly what you did before your surgery. You'll automatically push the covers away or just roll over into a different position. For more comfortable sleeping, keep the room adequately humidified and avoid fuzzy bedding that may release fibers that cause you to cough.

◆ If a "Neck Breather" Has a Medical Emergency

It will be important that you, your family, and others are aware of emergency procedures if you should have a respiratory arrest or another type of medical emergency. When you have a permanent tracheostomy, no air passes through the nose or mouth. In simple terms, you are a "neck breather." During medical emergencies, it is useless to try mouth-to-mouth breathing in any individual who breathes through an opening in the neck. It is necessary to use mouth-to-stoma rescue breathing or a variation of this technique with a barrier device. *For current information on rescue breathing techniques and procedures for persons with a tracheostomy, contact the American Red Cross or the International Association of Laryngectomees.* Wear an emergency medical bracelet that identifies you as a neck breather. Some people carry a brightly colored emergency card in their pocket to identify themselves as a neck breather. Consider notifying your local police, fire department, and medical emergency personnel that you are a neck breather and that if you have a medical emergency, you may be unable to speak.

G

Posture Training and Upper Body Exercises after Treatments for Cancer of the Head and Neck

◆ Posture, Mobility, and Strength are Usually Affected

Surgery, radiation therapy, and chemotherapy for head and neck cancer affect nerves and muscles in the neck, shoulders, chest, and arms. As a result, normal posture, mobility, and strength are usually affected. Your shoulder (or shoulders) may droop, and you may have a tendency to move your head and trunk together rather than using natural head movements. Ask your physician if the following activity suggestions are appropriate for you.

◆ Suggestions for Posture and Participation in Activities

- Maintain good posture by keeping your shoulders back and relaxed and your chin slightly tucked in. Good posture prevents the chest muscles from pulling against the weaker muscles on the back of your shoulder. Good posture also prevents extra pressure and minimizes discomfort. To increase your awareness of shoulder positioning, stand in front of a large mirror to see if you are aligning your shoulders evenly. Follow this by attempting to align your shoulders evenly with your eyes closed. Then open your eyes to check your posture.
- Avoid sitting or standing to the point of discomfort. This prevents tiring muscles that maintain good posture. When sitting, try to sit in a chair with a straight back. If this is not possible, put a pillow behind your back for support. Lie down occasionally during the day for short periods. You will need less rest as you begin to feel better.
- Lie on your back when sleeping. Try putting a small pillow under your spine between your shoulder blades and a pillow under your neck. Sleeping on your side may promote the posture you are trying to prevent. If you must lie on your side, lie on your uninvolved or less involved side and put your involved arm on the side of your body with your elbow bent and your hand supported on a pillow.

- Wear an arm support, if one has been prescribed, when you are sitting, standing, or walking, especially during the early weeks after surgery. If it is not possible to wear the support, protect your involved arm by placing your uninvolved hand under the elbow of the involved arm and gently prop up the elbow.
- Support your involved arm and hand on a desk, the arm of a chair, or a pillow whenever you are reading or writing. Put your hand on your hip to relieve the weight whenever necessary.
- Avoid using your involved arm to lift or carry objects of any weight until you can do so without discomfort. Heavier objects can cause damage and increase pain in your shoulder. Do not carry shoulder bags or purses on your involved side until you can do so without discomfort.
- Do not bend your head backward as if looking up to the ceiling until you can do so without discomfort. If you can, use a straw for drinking rather than pulling your head backward to drink from a glass.
- Everyday routines can help you regain strength. Think of the movements involved in combing your hair, drying after bathing, cooking, folding clothes, vacuuming, driving, and gardening. Remember to take it easy at first, and increase the activity step by step.

The restricting activities listed above and the following exercises may be discontinued when your mobility and strength become more normal and you feel you are no longer benefiting from these suggestions.

◆ Important Points to Remember about Exercising

The following exercises are designed to speed your recovery after head and neck cancer treatments. Your physical therapist will show you how to do each exercise. The physical therapist will indicate only the exercises recommended for you and will help you determine the number of times to repeat each exercise and how often to do it each day. If you have any questions after you get home, please call your physical therapist or physician.

- Do the recommended exercises only in the position shown.
- Avoid fast and jerky movements.
- Keep your head in line with your neck and shoulders throughout the exercise routine. Straighten your neck so that the top of your head reaches toward the ceiling. Tuck in your chin slightly and keep you shoulders relaxed. This posture prevents the chest muscles from tightening and pulling against the weaker muscles of the neck and shoulder.
- After every third, fifth, and tenth repetition, take one long deep breath, as described in Diaphragmatic Breathing and Pursed Lip Breathing, below. Breathing exercises can also be done while you sit or stand. If you have had a tracheostomy, you should still breathe deeply. This deep breathing routine may help decrease muscle spasms, which may ease discomfort.
- Do not exercise past the point of discomfort.

◆ Neck Exercises

Do not put a pillow under head when you lie down to exercise. Keep your knees bent and your feet flat when you lie on your back.

Lie on your _____ side, facing straight ahead. Rest your head on your bent arm. Make sure your head is aligned with your neck and shoulders. Bend your chin to your chest. Repeat this movement _____ times. Do _____ times a day (Fig. G–1).

Lie on your back, looking at the ceiling. Turn your head to the right, then the left. Move your head as far as possible in each direction. Repeat this movement _____ times. Do _____ times a day (Fig. G–2).

Lie on your back. Keeping your shoulders down and resting on the surface, try to touch your left ear to your left shoulder. Then try to touch your right ear to your right shoulder. Do not shrug your shoulders. Repeat this movement _____ times. Do _____ times a day (Fig. G–3).

◆ Shoulder Exercises

Lie on your back. Your arms should rest at your sides and your head should be lined up with your neck and shoulders. Keep your chin slightly tucked in toward your neck. Inhale slowly while drawing your shoulders slowly upward. Hold this position for a count of _____ . Avoid pain. Exhale slowly as you gradually relax the muscles of your neck and upper back and return to your original position. Rest between repetitions. Repeat this movement _____ times. Do _____ times a day (Fig. G–4).

Lie on your back with your _____ arm at your side. Slowly raise your arm up toward the ceiling and then up along the side of your head as far as possible. Return your arm to its starting position in the other direction. Keep your elbow straight throughout the motion. Use your other hand to help, if necessary. Repeat this movement _____ times. Do _____ times a day (Fig. G–5).

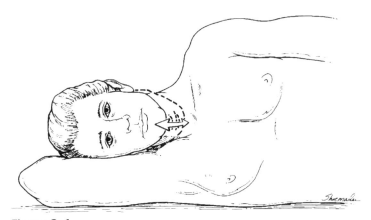

Figure G–1

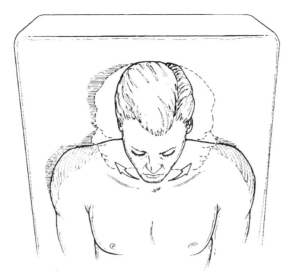

Figure G–2

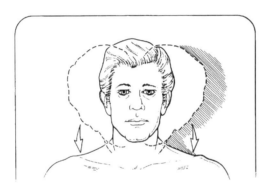

Figure G–3

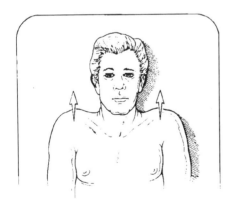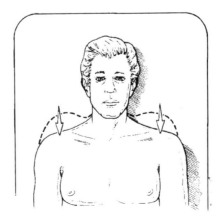

Figure G–4

Lie on your back with your _____ arm at your side. Move your arm out to the side and then up next to your head as far as possible, without raising it off the surface. Return your arm to its starting position. Keep your elbow straight at all times. Repeat this movement _____ times. Do _____ times a day (Fig. G–6).

Lie on your back with your _____ arm at a right angle to your side and your elbow bent 90 degrees. Slowly roll your arm forward until the palm of your hand rests on the surface near your waist. Keep your elbow at shoulder level. Return your arm to its starting position. Slowly roll your arm backward until the back of your hand rests on the surface near your head. Return your arm to its starting position. Repeat this movement _____ times. Do _____ times a day (Fig. G–7).

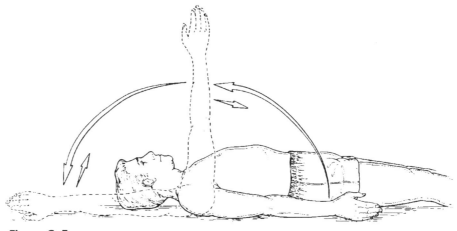

Figure G–5

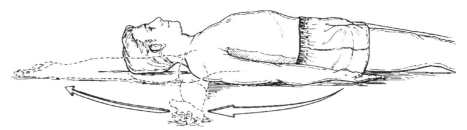

Figure G–6

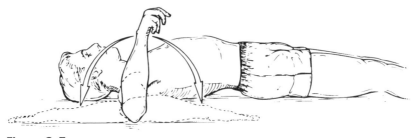

Figure G–7

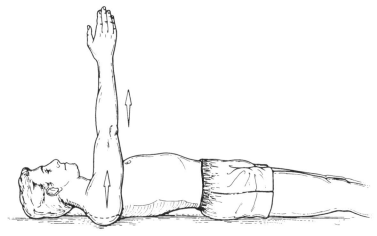

Figure G–8

Lie on your back with your _____ arm straight up and your fingers pointed at the ceiling. Reach toward the ceiling as far as possible. Then relax so the shoulder is resting back on the surface. Keep your elbow straight at all times. Repeat this movement _____ times. Do _____ times a day (Fig. G–8).

◆ Chest Muscle Stretches

Lie on your back with your knees bent. Put a rolled-up towel between your shoulder blades. For a stronger stretch, clasp your hands behind your neck, letting your elbow fall toward the surface. Hold for _____ , then relax. Repeat this movement _____ times. Do _____ times a day (Fig. G–9).

Stand facing the corner of a room. With your arms at shoulder level and feet shoulder-width apart, put one hand on each wall. Bend your elbows, keeping your back straight. Your fingers should point toward the corner.

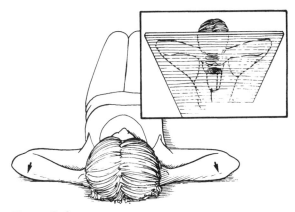

Figure G–9

Slowly let the weight of your body go forward, moving your chest toward the corner. Hold for _____ , then relax. Repeat this movement _____ times. Do _____ times a day (Fig. G–10).

◆ Neck Exercises with Wall Support

Sit in a straight-backed chair with its back against a wall. With your arm supported at your side, repeat exercises (Figs. G–1, G–2, G–3, and G–7). Rest your head against the wall. This exercise may also be done while standing with your back and head against a wall. Repeat this movement _____ times. Do _____ times a day.

◆ Neck Exercises without Support

Sit in a straight-backed chair or stand against a wall without your head supported. Repeat exercises (Figs. G–1, G–2, G–3, and G–7). Repeat this movement _____ times. Do _____ times a day.

◆ Shoulder and Arm Exercises against Gravity

Sit in a straight-backed chair or stand against a wall. Repeat exercises (Figs. G–4, G–5, and G–6). Repeat this movement _____ times. Do _____ times a day.

◆ Shoulder Blade Exercise

Sit or stand with arms at your side. Squeeze your shoulder blades together as tight as possible. Hold for _____ seconds, then release. Repeat this movement _____ times. Do _____ times a day (Fig. G–11).

◆ Arm Exercises

Put the hand from your involved side behind your neck. Move your arm down your back as far as possible. Keep your head lined up with your neck and shoulders as described earlier. Repeat this movement _____ times. Do this _____ times a day (Fig. G–12).

Put the hand from your involved side behind your waist. Move your arm up your back as far as possible. Repeat this movement _____ times. Do _____ times a day (Fig. G–13).

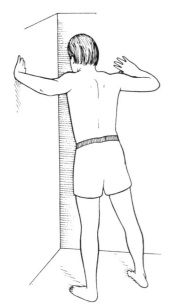

Figure G–10

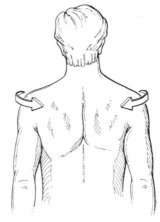

Figure G–11

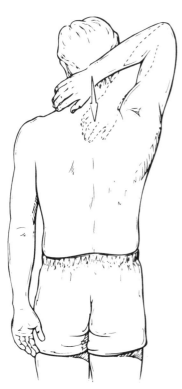

Figure G–12

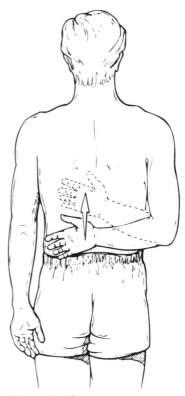

Figure G–13

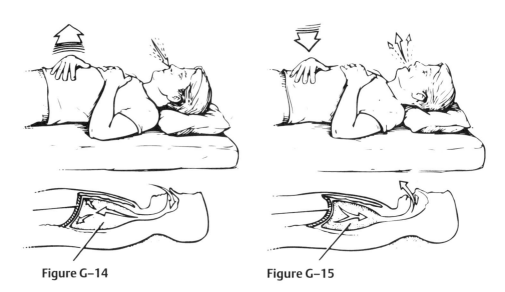

Figure G–14   Figure G–15

◆ Diaphragmatic Breathing and Pursed Lip Breathing

Breathing exercises develop a breathing pattern that will help you recover your breath sooner and easier whenever you get out of breath. Breathing exercises do not change or improve the lungs themselves. But when you breathe according to these instructions, the exercises may help the lungs work more efficiently. Practice is necessary before you will be able to breathe this way comfortably. *Diaphragmatic breathing* can be practiced while you are lying down, sitting, or standing.

Lie on your back with your head slightly raised on a pillow. Place one hand on your abdomen and one on your chest. Inhale through your nose or tracheostomy, expanding your abdomen. Do not move the upper chest (Fig. G–14). Now, exhale (breathe out) through your mouth or tracheostomy. As you exhale, contract our abdominal muscles to push the air out of your lungs. Don't force the air out. Take at least two to three times as long for exhaling as for inhaling. Practice until you can breathe comfortably in this manner (Fig. G–15).

If you do not have a tracheostomy, use pursed lip breathing with the diaphragmatic breathing technique, but only when you exhale. As you exhale, pucker or purse your lips. This will produce a gentle resistance to the outflow of air. Notice that your abdomen moves up when you inhale and moves down when you exhale. Pursed lip breathing can be used whenever you are short of breath. This may include when you are standing, walking, or climbing stairs.

◆ Acknowledgment

Appendix G is reprinted from an educational booklet titled *Home Instruction after Head and Neck Surgery* by A. Schutt, 1991, Rochester, MN: Mayo Clinic.

H

Sources of Information and Support

◆ Sources of Reliable Medical Information

Everything changes. Company names, business owners, addresses, telephone and fax numbers, Web sites, and e-mail addresses change all the time. Rather than provide names and addresses of medical institutions, support organizations, sources of information, or vendors of products, we suggest you go to the Internet and look up general categories such as "laryngectomy," "glossectomy," or "head and neck cancer." There are inherent drawbacks in this approach, as the warning below describes; however, there are some excellent starting places on the Internet for reliable medical information:

- *MayoClinic.com*
- *cancer.gov* (National Cancer Institute)
- American Cancer Society
- International Association of Laryngectomees (IAL)

These organizations and others have excellent pamphlets and other printed information available on cancer, statistics, types of treatment, outcomes, and much more.

◆ Searching for Information

- If you have had a total laryngectomy, visit the Web site of the *International Association of Laryngectomees* (also known as IAL) for current listings of postlaryngectomy equipment, vendors, services, and information on aspects of life after total laryngectomy.
- Search the Internet with other key words such as the name of a specific piece of equipment or treatment. Examples: *artificial larynx* or *radiation therapy*. Most public libraries have access to the Internet. Ask for assistance, if needed.
- Look through your telephone directory for the branch of the American Cancer Society near you. If the branch cannot help you, it may have suggestions on where to search for the information you need.
- For questions about speech, voice, and swallowing, contact a speech pathologist in a hospital or medical center or contact the speech-language-hearing association in your state. If you are unable to locate the organization

in your state, contact the American Speech-Language-Hearing Association (ASHA) or go to the ASHA Web site at *www.asha.com.*

- Ask your physician or caregiver for printed information about your condition or ask for recommendations of where to look.
- *Coping with Cancer* magazine is an excellent source of information and support. Often it can be found in the waiting areas of cancer treatment facilities.

◆ Be Cautious about...

Be cautious about medical information you locate on the Internet and anywhere else, particularly if you are not familiar with the source. Ask yourself, "Is the source of this information credible?" Ask the opinion of your family physician or a health care professional. The old adage, "If it sounds too good to be true, it probably is," applies to most circumstances in life, including dealing with cancer. Again, take the information you find to the physician who has examined you and knows your circumstances. For whatever reason, if you and your cancer specialist are not a good match, ask your family physician for recommendations on seeking a second opinion.

Finally, much of what you hear on talk shows and read in the popular press may not pertain to you and your exact medical condition. Avoid self-diagnosis and treatment.

Six Tips for Better Communication after Treatments for Cancer of the Larynx or Tongue

These suggestions are simple and they make sense. Practice them every day to become the best communicator you can be.

1. To get people's attention, say their name or do something so they are looking at you before you start speaking.
2. Be close and face-to-face when you speak to someone.
3. Eliminate as much noise in the environment as possible before you speak. If you do not recognize the disrupting noise in the background and do something about it, you will probably end up repeating yourself, or your listener will pretend to understand what you are saying or will understand only part of what you are saying. You must turn down the television or music. Turn off fans, noisy appliances, running water, etc. If it is noisy in the next room, shut the door. Move to a quieter place. Do whatever is necessary to make the environment the best for you to communicate in. If you do not do something to reduce the noise, no one will.
4. When you speak, think about "sending" your speech directly over to your listeners. Be determined that they *will* understand what you are saying.
5. When you are in a conversation or you are resuming a conversation, give the other person a signal that you are changing the topic of conversation.
6. Be patient with your listener. Be patient with yourself.

J

Communication Charts

MIRROR

COMB / BRUSH

CLOTHES

EYEGLASSES

PAPER & PEN

WHAT TIME IS IT?

BOOK / MAGAZINE

LIGHT ON / OFF

RADIO ON / OFF

TV ON / OFF

A	B	C	D	E	F	G
H	I	J	K	L	M	
N	O	P	Q	R	S	T
U	V	W	X	Y	Z	

0	1	2	3	4
5	6	7	8	9

10 20 30 40 50 100

Figure J–1 InHealth letter/word communication charts. (Courtesy of InHealth Technologies, Carpinteria, California. *www.inhealth.com.*)

Laryngectomy Needs Chart

CALL NURSE	NAUSEOUS
PAIN	MEDICATION
CONSTIPATION	DIARRHEA
IRRIGATE	SUCTION
CLEAN STOMA	BATH
BATHROOM	I AM COLD / HOT
CHANGE BED	BED PAN
DRY MOUTH	WATER
HUNGRY	JUICE
IN / OUT BED	ADJUST BED
TISSUE	WASHCLOTH

Figure J–1   (Continued)

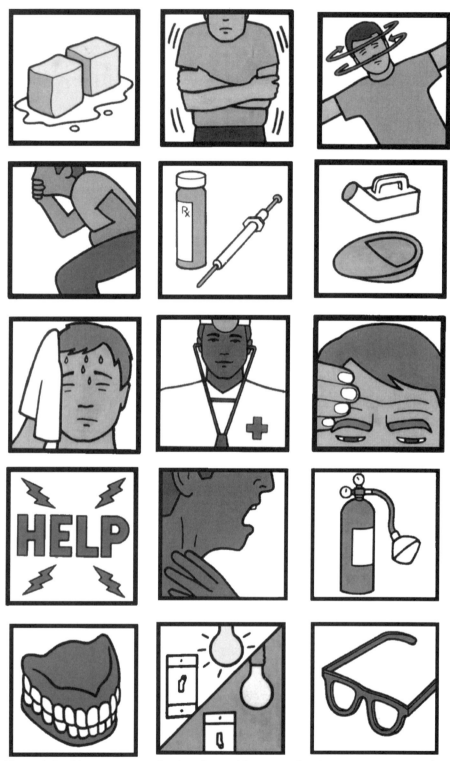

Figure J–2   Picture communication charts. (Courtesy of PRO-ED Inc. International, Austin, Texas.)

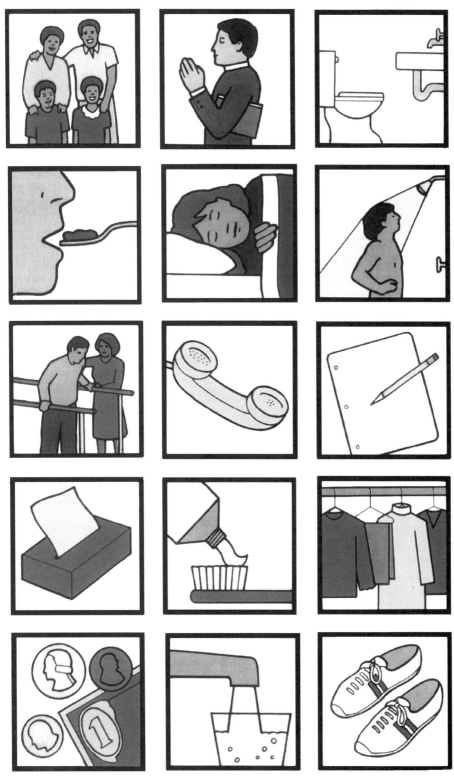

Figure J–2 (Continued)

Glossary

The purpose of this glossary is to acquaint you with some of the words that are often used by health care professionals concerning head and neck cancer and treatments for it. For some terms, you are directed to specific sections in *Looking Forward . . .* where the words are used and defined further. Also, when you read a word written in *italics*, it is defined in this glossary. Knowing these words will help in discussions you have with your medical team and help you better understand what you read about cancer, radiation therapy, chemotherapy, and surgery. Keep in mind that these are only some of the words you will hear and read concerning cancer of the larynx, tongue, and related topics. Ask your physician and other medical team members when they use a word that is unfamiliar to you.

Alaryngeal: Without a larynx or "voice box."

Artificial larynx: A manufactured instrument that makes a tone or "voice" which is used to produce speech after total laryngectomy (see Appendix B).

Aspiration: Breathing in food, liquid, or other material into the lungs (see Chapter 2 and Appendix D).

Biopsy: The removal of a sample of tissue for study under a microscope to determine if it contains cancer (Chapter 1).

Cannula: Part of a metal or plastic tube that is placed in the tracheostoma to keep it from closing. Some tubes have an outer cannula that acts as a sleeve for an inner cannula (see Chapter 7 and Appendix F).

Chemotherapy: A treatment for cancer using chemical agents. Chemotherapy is sometimes used in conjunction with radiation therapy and/or surgery (see Chapters 3 and 5).

Consistency: The degree of density, firmness, and texture of a liquid or food, such as a liquid with the consistency of nectar or honey (see Appendix D).

Cordectomy: Surgical removal of a vocal cord (see Chapter 6).

CT scan or CT scanning: An abbreviation for "computed axial tomography" or "computed tomography." A test using computers and x-rays to create images of various parts of the body (see Chapter 1).

Diaphragmatic breathing: A way to breathe deeply by relaxing the abdominal muscles to give the diaphragm more space to move down. This allows more air to enter the lungs. Tightening the abdominal muscles during exhalation pushes more air out (see Appendix G).

Dietitian: A professional who specializes in diet and nutrition.

Direct laryngoscopy: The use of an instrument with its own light source to enable a surgeon to look directly at the larynx. The instrument resembles a pipe and is usually used when a patient is under general anesthesia (see Chapter 1).

Dysphagia: Difficulty swallowing (see Appendix D).

Electrocautery: The application of electric current to destroy tissue.

ENT or otorhinolaryngologist: A physician who specializes in diseases of the ears, nose, and throat, and head and neck cancer (see Chapter 1).

Enteral feeding: Receiving food through a tube (see Appendix C).

Epiglottis: A lidlike structure made of cartilage that tilts down to protect the larynx during swallowing (see Chapter 2).

Esophageal voice or esophageal speech: A method of speaking after the entire larynx has been surgically removed (total laryngectomy). To produce esophageal voice, air is intentionally trapped in the upper esophagus. It produces a sound or "voice" when it is released into the pharynx and mouth where it is shaped into speech by the lips, tongue, teeth, and hard and soft palates. The terms *esophageal voice* and *esophageal speech* are often used interchangeably (see Appendix B).

Esophagus: The passageway or "tube" that takes food and liquids from the throat down to the stomach (see Chapter 2).

Exhalation: The part of respiration when you breathe out (see Appendix G).

False vocal folds or false vocal cords: Protective valves of the larynx that prevent food and liquids from entering the trachea.

Fiberoptic endoscopic evaluation of swallowing and sensory testing (FEESST): A method of examining a person's swallowing ability and sensation using a flexible endoscope inserted through the nose (see Appendix D).

Fiberoptic laryngoscope: A flexible instrument used to examine the nasal, oral (mouth), pharyngeal (throat), and laryngeal (vocal folds) passages.

Fiberoptic laryngoscopy: Examination of the larynx and related areas using a fiberoptic, flexible endoscope (see Chapter 1).

Fine-needle aspiration: A procedure to remove cells or fluid from tissues using a needle with an empty syringe. Cells are extracted by pulling back on the plunger and then are analyzed by a physician (pathologist) (see Chapter 1).

Fine-needle biopsy: A procedure in which a needle is inserted under local anesthesia to obtain a sample for the examination of suspicious tissue (see Chapter 1).

Fistula: An opening along a surgical incision that causes food or saliva to drain to the outside. A fistula may be a sign of incomplete healing (see Chapter 6).

Forearm free flap: A flap of tissue and vessels moved from the forearm, rolled into a tube, and used to reconstruct the pharynx (see Chapter 6).

Free flap: Healthy tissue from one part of the body that is used to reconstruct a part that has been surgically removed due to cancer, such as skin and muscle removed from the forearm or chest that is rolled into a tube and used to reconstruct the pharynx (see Chapters 6 and 7).

Gastric pull-up: A method of reconstruction when the pharynx (throat) and esophagus are removed due to cancer. The stomach is "pulled up" to take the place of the removed structures (see Chapter 6).

Glossectomy: Surgical removal of the tongue (see Chapter 7).

Glottic cancers: Cancer involving the vocal folds (cords).

Heat and moisture exchanger (HME): A filter placed over the tracheostoma after laryngectomy that captures heat and moisture when air is exhaled from the lungs, then returns the heat and moisture when air is inhaled (see Appendix F).

Hemiglossectomy: A surgical procedure to remove part of the tongue because of cancer (see Chapter 7).

Hemilaryngectomy: A surgical procedure to remove part of the larynx (voice box) usually because of cancer (see Chapter 6).

Indirect laryngoscopy: The use of light reflected from a mirror held in the back of the patient's mouth to examine the larynx (see Chapter 1).

Intelligible: The amount of speech that is understood by the listener; for example, "His speech was about 50% intelligible to his family members, but only about 25% intelligible to people who did not know him well."

International Association of Laryngectomees (IAL): An international organization run by laryngectomized people in many countries providing support and education to other laryngectomees (see Appendix H).

Jejunum: A section of the small intestine sometimes used in the reconstruction of the pharynx (see Chapter 6).

Laryngeal: Having to do with the larynx.

Laryngectomee: A person whose larynx has been removed (see Appendix B).

Laryngectomy: The surgical procedure to remove the larynx (see Chapter 6 and Appendices B and F).

Laryngoscope: An instrument used to examine the larynx (see Chapter 1).

Larynx: The organ of sound production; the vocal folds or cords; sometimes called the "voice box."

Laser: A surgical instrument that produces a powerful beam of light to vaporize (cancerous) tissue.

Linear accelerator: Equipment that delivers radiation therapy (see Chapter 4).

Lymph nodes: Rounded bodies of lymph tissue that filter bacteria and other particles, including cancer cells, from the lymphatic system. They are part of the body's immune system (see Chapter 1).

Lymphedema: Swelling due to poor lymphatic drainage (see Chapter 8).

Magnetic resonance imaging (MRI): A radiological test that provides in-depth images of organs and structures of the body (see Chapter 1).

Malignant tumor: A tumor made up of cancer cells of the type that can spread to other parts of the body.

Maxillofacial prosthodontist: A dentist with additional training who specializes in dental and facial restoration and reconstruction (see Chapters 3 and 7).

Metastatic: Cancer that spreads to other parts of the body.

Nasogastric (NG) tube: A flexible plastic tube that is introduced through the nostril and advanced to the stomach (see Chapter 6).

Near-total laryngectomy: Removal of most of the larynx including the vocal folds, except for a cancer-free part of one fold. This procedure preserves a voice, but a tracheostoma is necessary for breathing. The surgeon must determine if a person with cancer of the larynx is a candidate for this surgery (see Chapter 6).

Neck dissection: The surgical removal of lymph nodes and some surrounding structures within the neck (see Chapter 6).

Oncologist or medical oncologist: A physician who specializes in the study and treatment of cancer with cancer-fighting medicines called chemotherapy (see Chapter 5).

Oropharynx: The area behind the tongue at the back of the throat. This area can be seen through the mouth (see Chapter 2).

Otolaryngologist: Physician specializing in otolaryngology.

Palatal augmentation prosthesis: A plastic-like device that fits up close to the roof of the mouth (palate) to lower it. A palatal augmentation prosthesis is sometimes created for a person who has had much or most of the tongue surgically removed. It may allow the remaining or reconstructed tongue to contact it to aid in swallowing and production of speech sounds (see Chapter 7).

Palliative: Treatment intended not to cure cancer but to control its growth, reduce complications, and alleviate pain or other symptoms related to cancer growth (see Chapter 5).

Partial glossectomy: A surgery to remove part of the tongue (see Chapter 7).

Partial laryngectomy: A surgery to remove part of the larynx. There are many types of partial laryngectomy (see Chapter 6).

Pathologist: A medical doctor who specializes in identifying diseases by studying cells and tissues under a microscope.

Pectoral myocutaneous flap: Using the chest skin and muscle to reconstruct removed areas, such as in the throat or mouth.

Percutaneous endoscopic gastrostomy (PEG): A surgery to place a feeding tube into the stomach. The feeding tube may also be referred to as a PEG tube (see Appendix C).

Peripherally inserted central catheter (PICC): A thin, flexible tube placed in a vein of the arm to slowly administer medication, blood products, or nutritional supplements. A PICC is used to deliver some types of chemotherapy (see Chapter 5).

Pharyngo-laryngo-esophagectomy: A surgery to remove the pharynx (throat), larynx (voice box), and esophagus (food tube) (Chapter 6).

Pharynx: The medical term for the throat. The passage between the mouth and the larynx (voice box) and the esophagus (food tube) (see Chapter 2).

Pulmonary: Concerning breathing and the lungs.

Radiation oncologist: A physician who specializes in diagnosis of cancer and treating cancer with radiation therapy (see Chapter 4).

Radiation therapy: A method of destroying cancer cells. Radiation therapy is sometimes used in addition to or instead of surgery and/or chemotherapy. Also known as "radiation," "irradiation," "radiotherapy," and "x-ray therapy" (see Chapter 4).

Referred pain: The feeling of pain in an area distant from the cause of the pain but supplied by the same nerve. For example, ear pain can be referred from the larynx, even though there is no direct problem with the ear itself, because both the ear and the larynx are supplied by the same nerve (Chapter 1).

Speech pathologist: A professional specializing in speech, language, and swallowing disorders.

Stoma cover: A cloth or foam covering or biblike piece of material used to cover the tracheostoma to prevent dust or foreign matter from being inhaled. A stoma cover can help prevent clothing from being soiled by mucus. There are other benefits to wearing a stoma cover (see Appendix F).

Stoma or tracheostoma: A surgically created, permanent opening in the front of the neck. After total laryngectomy or near-total laryngectomy, air is inhaled and exhaled through the stoma, not through the mouth or nose (see Chapters 6 and 7, and Appendix F).

Supracricoid partial laryngectomy: Surgical removal of much of the larynx with preservation of parts of it to allow production of voice.

Supraglottic laryngectomy: Surgical removal of the upper parts of the larynx to the level immediately above the vocal cords (see Chapter 6).

Total glossectomy: Surgical removal of the entire tongue or the majority of it (see Chapter 7).

Total laryngectomy: A surgery to remove the entire larynx including the vocal folds (see Chapter 6 and Appendices B and F).

Trachea: The windpipe; the air passageway between the larynx and the lungs (see Chapter 1).

Tracheoesophageal puncture (TEP): A surgical procedure in which an opening is made between the trachea and the esophagus just behind the stoma. A voice prosthesis can then be placed in the tracheoesophageal puncture (see Chapter 6 and Appendix B).

Tracheoesophageal voice prosthesis or voice prosthesis: A silicone tube ~0.25 to 0.5 inch in length and smaller than the diameter of a pencil that is placed between the trachea and esophagus after total laryngectomy and tracheoesophageal puncture. The prosthesis is open on the tracheal end. It has a valve on the esophageal end that keeps foods and fluids from moving through the prosthesis and into the trachea and lungs. As the person exhales and covers the tracheostoma with a finger or thumb, air flows up through the lungs and through the prosthesis causing part of the upper esophagus to vibrate and produce sound. This sound is the "tracheoesophageal voice" that is shaped into speech by the tongue, lips, and other parts of the mouth (Chapter 6, Appendix B).

Tracheostoma: See *Stoma or tracheostoma.*

Tracheostomy: An opening into the trachea (windpipe) (see Chapter 6 and Appendices B and F).

Tracheostomy tube or trach tube: A metal or plastic tube inserted into the stoma to make early postoperative tracheostomy care easier and to prevent the stoma from shrinking (see Chapter 6 and Appendix F).

Transoral laser surgeries or transoral endoscopic surgeries: see Chapter 8.

True vocal folds or true vocal cords: See *vocal folds or vocal cords.*

Tumor: An abnormal overgrowth of cells. Tumors can be benign (noncancerous) or malignant (cancerous).

Videofluoroscopic swallow study or x-ray swallow study: Also referred to or related to "modified barium swallow test" and "videofluorographic swallow study." A test performed to identify which foods and liquids are easiest for a person to swallow and where in the swallowing mechanism there may be problems. The person swallows liquid barium and thicker barium mixed into small amounts of foods. The barium can be seen on the x-ray, and the movement of the material through the mouth and throat can be seen. This test can help determine changes in muscular activity in the mouth and throat and if foods and liquids are entering the lungs. If the person has had head and neck surgery, this test can help determine if there has been adequate healing (see Appendix D).

Vocal folds or vocal cords: Two small shelves of muscular tissue within the larynx. They vibrate against each other and generate sound known as "voice." They are part of the "valving system" that prevents food from entering the trachea and lungs (see Chapter 2).

Voice box: The common term for the larynx or vocal folds.

Voice prosthesis: See "tracheoesophageal voice prosthesis," above.

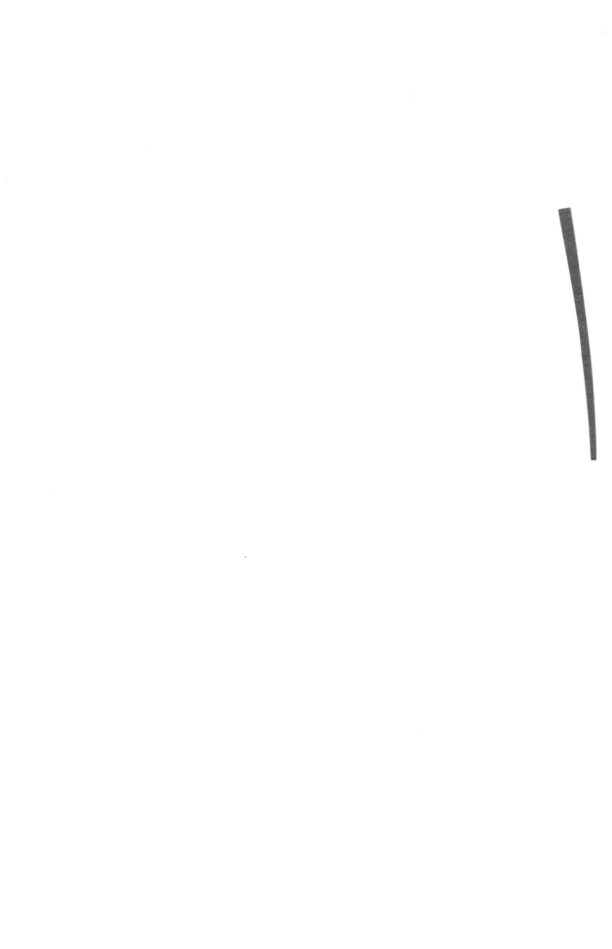